Personal Growth Through Crises

Gene Burnell

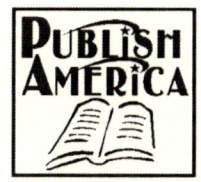

PublishAmerica
Baltimore

First printing

At the specific preference of the author, PublishAmerica allowed this work to remain exactly as the author intended, verbatim, without editorial input.

ISBN: 1-4241-5530-4
PUBLISHED BY PUBLISHAMERICA, LLLP
www.publishamerica.com
Baltimore

Printed in the United States of America

Dedication

This book is dedicated to my wife, Gwen, for her endless love and support through good times, but most of all through life's challenges. Our love has only grown deeper in the challenging times. And to my children, Todd, Garrett and Whitney, who have provided tremendous joy in my life.

Preface

First and foremost, I want everyone reading this book to know that I consider myself extremely blessed. For many years, I have been a cancer patient, but I am in remission at this time. Since 1993, my cancer has occurred five different times. Fortunately, each time my body has responded positively to treatments. Second and extremely important, my family is a tremendous support group, as well as the church congregation that I attend, long-time friends and my fellow employees. I am completely surrounded by loving people who care for me as husband, father, as a friend and as a fellow-worker. My most comforting influence, however, is my God, and knowing that with Him all things are possible. He has blessed me with a strong faith for which I am very grateful.

Some non-Hodgkin's lymphoma patients are not nearly so fortunate as I have been. They are stricken with a very aggressive form of cancer and their body does not respond positively to treatment. When I was first diagnosed with cancer in 1993, I had a combination of aggressive lymphoma and slow-growing lymphoma. The aggressive cancer did not return after my first round of chemotherapy treatments. Now in 2006, and celebrating thirteen years since my initial diagnosis of cancer, I have reached over five years in remission for the first time.

The purpose of my book is to share how those events, and many others, have impacted my life. In addition to explaining the impact of those events, I will share how I have dealt with those experiences and explain some of the lessons learned from them. My desire is that anyone reading this will find hope in the fact that someone else has faced these challenges and survived to be a better person.

I also want to acknowledge the web site, www.blueletterbible.com. All of my scriptures were found through their search engine. This tool has been very beneficial to my Bible study over the years.

Last, I want to express my sincere appreciation to our friend, Elaine, who proofed and edited my manuscript. Her ideas were a great improvement to my work.

Chapter 1

My "Wake-up" Call

It was a beautiful spring morning in Raleigh, North Carolina. I had spent the night with friends while on a business trip. While shaving, I noticed a raised, hardened mass under my chin, in the middle of my throat. It was early April 1993, and my rental car was dusted with yellow pollen spores from the vibrant foliage that had recently blossomed. My throat was swollen from allergies related to the pollen. I only noticed the lump, because my throat was enlarged. I continued to monitor the hard lump for about a month, before I told Gwen, my wife. When I showed it to her, I asked her to make me a doctor's appointment. I was very careful how I worded my request to see a doctor. I didn't want to alarm her. It seemed that Gwen was not really grasping what was being requested. She was not showing any emotion. The lump really concerned me. It had not changed in size or how it felt since I first noticed it, and that did not appear to be a good sign. In my mind, if it was nothing, it would have gone away.

Gwen made the appointment and a couple of weeks later I went to see the doctor. After poking around on the lump, and because of its location, he was "90 percent certain" that it was just a thyroid cyst and recommended me to a surgeon. The surgeon examined me and was also "90 percent" sure that it was just a thyroid cyst. My concerns were eased when both doctors appeared so confident. I was relieved to know that it was no big deal, or so it seemed. With my consent, the surgeon scheduled the surgery. He began discussing what to expect during my recuperation time following the surgery. The surgeon told me that I would miss about nine days work, and then I would be back on the job. Concerns dismissed and my wife at my side, I went to the hospital for minor surgery—removal of a thyroid cyst. I was entering the hospital as a patient for the first time in my life. The nurses joked with me, because I had such a short medical history. They said dealing with me was like dealing with a baby. They were impressed with my low blood pressure, low cholesterol levels and overall good health. When the time came, they wheeled me into the operating room. Immediately following the surgery, the doctor had some startling news for Gwen. He introduced himself, and asked Gwen if she had anyone with her. She explained that we had just moved into town and she was alone. He said something to the effect, "It was not what I expected, but we cleaned up the area very nicely and Gene is doing well. It was a lymph node and the tissue color was not what I anticipated." Because of his years of experience, he was familiar with what cancer looked like and he was trying to break the news to Gwen. He realized that she was not catching on to what he was implying, and again said, "Gene is doing very well but I think he is going to need some chemo." At that point, Gwen understood what he had been trying to tell her. He then told her that from his experience, he felt it was cancer, but that the tumor would be sent off for testing. That would be the final determination. It was in that moment that our lives changed. At that time, my oldest son was twelve, the younger son was ten and my daughter was eight.

Gwen had a huge burden on her shoulders knowing that I probably had cancer. She came into the recovery room to be with me. She said I responded to her with, "How did things go?" As delicately as possible, she tried to break the news to me that it was more serious than a cyst removal. The effects of the anesthesia were just starting to wear off, so I was not clear headed enough to handle the news at that time. We were soon discharged and returned home.

Some very good friends from Broken Arrow, Oklahoma, Wilson and Bobbie, were scheduled to arrive that afternoon for a weekend visit. They had scheduled their trip several months earlier. Gwen and I were excited that they were coming, and we did not want anything to delay their trip. We made sure that we did not tell them about my surgery out of fear that they would cancel their visit. They arrived shortly after Gwen and I returned from the hospital. When they arrived, it was obvious that I had just had surgery, because of the huge gauze pad taped to my neck. They said that this was probably not a good time, and volunteered to get a room at a hotel. We insisted that they stay at our house. I assured them that it was just a little outpatient surgery, and I would be fine. We did not know just how important it was that they did come to our house when we intentionally did not inform them of my surgery.

Our friends provided tremendous support for Gwen during their visit—someone who understood Gwen, but were not family members. Gwen did not have anyone in Texas to turn to for support. Six months earlier I had uprooted our family and moved from Oklahoma to Texas. We had just made a major lifestyle change by moving to an area where we did not know anyone. It was a true blessing that our friends were visiting us that particular weekend. Several times that evening, Gwen had heard me mention "that nothing was wrong and I was doing fine." She knew that she had told me about the cancer while I was in the recovery room, but it was becoming obvious that I didn't "get the message." Once she realized this, she wanted to tell me before our friends left town. She discussed the situation with Wilson and Bobbie, so they knew about it before me. Gwen was trying to decide when would be the right time to break the news to me. She knew that Wilson and Bobbie could provide some much needed support. We had attended church with them for many years in Tulsa and were very close. Wilson and Gwen had spent many hours together in Bible study when we lived in Oklahoma, and he was one of her dearest friends. They offered such wisdom, strength and faith, which was what Gwen needed right then. Since we were such close friends, we could be very frank in our conversations. On Sunday, Gwen told me, as delicately as she knew how, what the surgeon predicted. The test results were not available, but Gwen assured me that the doctor was convinced that it was cancer and I would need some chemotherapy. It is an understatement to say that the news was shocking to me. When I scheduled my surgery, cancer was not a possibility in my mind. Wilson and Bobbie extended their stay until Monday evening. We discussed the possibility of my having cancer at different times during their stay. When they left, I assured them that I was going to beat the cancer if it was indeed a reality. I was past the point of shock and pity. I was ready to face the challenges ahead. My quick mental turn around, was in part due to my competitive nature, and partly due to the discussions Gwen and I were able to have with our friends. I believe that you must face your health problems rather than deny them. Try to talk openly about your disease or illness. Accepting the fact that "my cancer was real" was very important for me. The sooner you accept it, the sooner you will be mentally prepared to fight it.

My scheduled follow-up appointment with the surgeon to let him check the stitches and to receive the test results was the next day, Tuesday. Soon after we arrived for my appointment, the nurse placed us in an examination room. During the wait, I was hopeful that the surgeon was wrong about the tissue that he had removed. I prayed to God that I did not have cancer. In my mind, there was still a chance that the lab reports would contradict my doctor's initial opinion.

Another few minutes passed, then he entered the exam room with a very troubled look on his face. He voiced a short, "Good afternoon!" but his expression was quite serious. He sat down by me, and got right to the point. He bluntly stated, "They have found cancer. Reports show that you have Hodgkin's disease." It was the only way that he knew to deliver such a bleak message. He was an extremely caring individual, and I could tell that it was not easy for him.

A diagnosis of cancer—that was a devastating time when the surgeon informed us that I definitely had cancer. I was thirty-nine years old and thought that I was in great shape. I was feeling extremely healthy, and he was telling me that my biopsy results confirmed that I had cancer! You talk about a "wake up" call. Geez! I had not been sick for years. I felt great. I was running one to two miles, three to five nights a week. But, the facts could not be denied! I had cancer. The only question was, "How far had it spread?" I started thinking about my family's future—the life insurance that I had never got around to purchasing, and knowing that no one was going to sell it to me now. Questions started running through my head. "If I were to die, how would my family survive financially?" I never thought that this would happen to me, mainly because I had never smoked, drank alcohol or done anything to harm my body. My next thoughts were: "What about our kids? How were they going to react to this news?" I sure did not want them to be overly burdened. I knew that I felt fine and that I was not going to give up on life. Another question was, "How am I going to tell my parents? This is going to hit them hard." I was the baby of the family—thirty-nine, but still the baby.

That devastation from learning that I had cancer only lasted a few days. I was soon determined to fight the cancer for myself and for my family. I was not going to mope around the house, or give up and expect the worst. Instead, I was determined that I would do everything I could to beat the dreaded disease. My first treatment was still a few weeks away, so I continued to jog. I was committed to being in the best possible physical condition when treatments were started. Once I started treatments, Gwen and I continued to walk in the evenings. I did all I could to keep my body as strong as possible.

During that follow-up appointment, the surgeon recommended an oncology group for us to consider. We made an appointment to see one of the oncologists in that group. The earliest appointment time that they had was a week away. Waiting was the worst part. The last thing I wanted to be doing was "nothing." I wanted to go to the oncologist the next day. I did not want to wait around and let the cancer grow and grow. In my estimation, it needed to be removed immediately! The surgeon had told me that I had cancer growing inside of me, and I wanted to get it out of there as soon as possible. When we finally saw the oncologist, he started explaining that they would be treating me for non-Hodgkin's lymphoma. Gwen and I quickly corrected the oncologist, telling him that the report that my surgeon read stated that I had Hodgkin's disease. However, between the time that my surgeon informed me of my initial diagnosis and my first visit with the oncologist, a revised pathology report had been issued. Upon further examination of the biopsy, my diagnosis had changed from Hodgkin's disease to non-Hodgkin's lymphoma. That was very unsettling to Gwen and me, because we had done our own research on the side. Through that research, we had learned that Hodgkin's disease was difficult to treat, but it could be cured. On the other hand, we knew that non-Hodgkin's lymphoma was treatable, but not curable. My initial thought was that out of those two possibilities, I was glad that I had Hodgkin's disease. Then I found out that I did not have Hodgkin's! We had prepared for one thing. Now we had to face something that we considered to be much worse.

Before the oncologist could recommend a series of treatments, he needed to know the extent of the cancer. The oncologist called the hospital and scheduled me for a full series of CT scans to make his determination. I had never had a CT scan before. Little did I know that would just be the first of many CT scans in my life. I have averaged far more than one CT scan a year for the last 13 years. Each time my cancer recurred, I had a CT scan prior to beginning treatments, then one following the treatments. The scans were used to determine the extent of the cancer, and the effectiveness of the treatments. CT scans are my friend today. The doctors have monitored my cancer with great accuracy using the results of the scans. CT scans are relatively painless. Here is the sequence of steps leading up to and including the scans. First, the oncologist's office makes an appointment at the local hospital or imaging center. Next, I call the hospital for pre-admission registration a day or two before the procedure. I am not allowed to eat anything after midnight on the day before. Once they locate my admission paperwork, they inform the X-ray technicians that I am ready for the scan. In preparation for the scan, I have to drink a 44-ounce drink that contains trace materials for the scan. It is necessary to drink that within twenty minutes. The drink has a lemonade flavor, so it does not taste bad. After another twenty minutes, I am called into the CT scan area and I have to change into a gown. Once I have changed, they take me into the CT scan unit and position me. The technician runs a few test scans to get me properly aligned on the table. Then I am given an IV (intravenous injection) of another trace material. That injection causes me to have a very metallic taste in my mouth, but that taste only lasts for a few minutes. The scans of my neck, chest and abdomen are completed within five minutes now. Ten years ago it would take up to 45 minutes. The new scanning equipment is much faster. For me, the scan does not cause me to be claustrophobic. The table on which you lay moves through a doughnut shaped X-ray unit that is only about twelve inches deep, so you don't feel trapped at all. A CT-scan is nothing to fear.

I was anxious to have my first CT scans, but the hospital was not able to schedule an appointment for me immediately. More days passed without any treatment. After the CT scans were completed, it took another five to seven days for the oncologist to receive the results. Again, the waiting was the worst part. I did not want to worry about the cancer. I was maintaining a positive attitude, but there was no way that I could just put it out of my mind. I had never experienced anything like that before. My thoughts were, "How fast is this cancer growing? How critical is each day in fighting it?" Of course, they could not begin treatments until they knew the extent of the disease inside my body. I knew that, but at the same time, I wanted treatment to start. But how do they know what treatment should be used? The waiting was necessary, but not pleasant.

The day of the appointment to receive the CT scan results finally arrived. The doctor began to review the results with us. We were shocked when he told us that I had stage III cancer. We had already done enough research to know that the severity of cancer was divided into four stages, with stage IV being the worst. As healthy as I felt, I was certain that I would only have stage I of the disease. For me to be at stage III and experiencing zero side effects from the cancer was puzzling. My oncologist explained that if the disease is above and below your diaphragm, it is automatically a stage III disease, even though all of the nodules were relatively small. I was very fortunate to not be experiencing any ill-effects, but it was still shocking to hear that I could be that far along. That meant that I had cancer throughout my body, and that was scary. We kind of laughed it off saying, "That shouldn't surprise us. It wasn't supposed to be cancer either! It was just a cyst." The oncologist also discussed his philosophy about predicting the

14

results of the treatments and declaring someone terminally ill. He said, "I will never tell anyone that they only have six months or a year to live. Patients just love it when a doctor tells them that they only have a short time to live and they live a lot longer. Patients are quick to point out how wrong the doctor was in making that assessment." Further, he stated that if their life ended much sooner than he said, it was very disappointing to the patient's family. Next, the oncologist elaborated on the treatments that would be used to treat my cancer and what I should be expecting. He referred to the treatment as CHOP. CHOP is a treatment, which consists of Cyclophosphamide, Vincristine (Oncovintin is the trade name for Vincristine), Adriamiacin and Prednizone. He made it clear that I would lose my hair and explained some of the possible side-effects that we needed to understand. The Adriamiacin can be very damaging to the heart and I was told to be sure and warn them if I noticed any pains, weaknesses, etc. In an attempt to provide some comfort, he stated that any medical intern would know the proper treatment for my type of cancer, because the treatment for non-Hodgkin's lymphoma had not changed in over twenty years.

Finally we had some answers! This may sound a little crazy, but I was relieved to know what I was dealing with and to know how it would be treated, and most importantly, that treatments were going to start! It was going to be difficult, but the alternative was worse. At least three weeks had passed since surgery. In my mind, precious time was getting away from us! While the oncologist was explaining the treatment process, he warned us of many potential challenges ahead. One was that I would probably need to be hospitalized two or three times, because my white blood cell counts would go dangerously low about two weeks after a treatment.

Eight treatments were prescribed. My treatments were scheduled every three weeks. On the first day of a treatment, I was given three injections of different drugs via an intravenous injection (IV). I was required to take Prednizone pills, a steroid, for the next ten days. I was told that Prednizone was lethal to lymphoma. Dosage levels were high to start, but decreased each day. My body responded to that steroid as if I had received a huge blast of energy. That gave me a better understanding of the phrase, "he must be on 'roids." I was so restless that I was looking for things to do, and that was not normal for me. I can usually sit down in an easy chair and relax, forgetting most anything. But the Prednizone had me zooming. I could not sleep much, maybe three to four hours a night, then I'd be up anxious to go. Some days I went into work early. Other times, Gwen would awaken in the middle of the night, because she heard a noise, would see lights on downstairs, or noticed I was missing from the bedroom. She would come downstairs to see what I was doing, or just called out, "Are you okay?" Sometimes, I would be cleaning the house, doing dishes or sweeping the floor. This was also when my journaling and note writing started. At one point, I generated a list of catchy phrases (related to cancer treatment and its side effects) for t-shirts, but I never carried out the idea. Two days after my last dose of the steroid, there was a significant difference. There was no longer that burst of energy. I became very tired by the end of the workday. Sleeping was not a problem. My temperament also changed. I became very short tempered, which is foreign to my laid back personality. Gwen warned the kids each time that I began reducing the dosage. They were young and my personality change was shocking at times. Some of my actions were puzzling to me. The positive and negative side effects of taking Prednizone repeated itself after each treatment was administered. My oncologist had warned us that it could cause me to become 'mean'. Gwen was always on the lookout for this.

Two weeks after my first chemotherapy treatment, my hair started falling out in globs. I decided to have some fun with my hair. I went through a couple of stages. First, I had Gwen shave the edges and cut the top very short. We went out on the back porch with the hair clippers and Gwen "fashioned" my hair, while our dog, Shadow, watched. As my hair loss progressed, the next stage was shaving my head clean. There was one particular morning when the reality of me taking chemotherapy and the affects that it would have on me really struck Gwen. She was asleep in bed. I had gotten up much earlier to get ready for work. She rolled over and grabbed my pillow as she had often done. This time was different, though. There was a huge glob of hair on the pillow. Later, she explained to me that was a very sobering moment for her, because she clearly recognized that I was in a battle for my life. Before, she had noticed thick clumps of hair in the trash where I had picked it up from the shower drain, but this was different. My hair loss was not just on my head either. I had grown a mustache, and I had a habit of twirling it as I sat around. One day I was twirling it, and the next thing I knew, I had a handful of whiskers. I looked in the mirror and I had a huge bald spot in my mustache. Did I mention that I was at work when this happened? That evening, it was time to shave it off. The kids and I had some fun removing it. They watched and laughed as I shaped the mustache like Hitler's. As time passed, I even lost most of my body hair. Years later, I learned that Gwen had kept a significant amount of my fallen hair in a zip-lock bag. She saved it for several years as a keepsake should I lose the battle. For her, it was a secret way of keeping a part of me.

While taking treatments, I had to be careful and avoid anyone who was dealing with anything contagious, particularly in the ten to fifteen days following a treatment. During that time, my white blood cell count was at its lowest level. White blood cells fight off infections, viruses, etc. They are critical to a strong immune system. I was fortunate, in that my white blood count never reached a seriously low level.

There was never any need for hospitalization—I was very fortunate.

The evening of my fifth treatment, I became very ill. After leaving the doctor's office, I went home and lay down on the couch as normal. A few hours later, the nausea started. That sickness lasted throughout the night and most of the next day. I did not feel good enough to go to work the next day. Things had gone smoothly the first four treatments. For the last four, I suffered one day of sickness each time and missed a total of four days of work. Gwen said that she watched me very closely when I was feeling badly. She remembers that one evening when she kissed me good night, she felt the heat from my lips, which indicated I had fever. That caused her to call the doctor.

One of the more amusing, yet tiresome, side effects that I suffered was severe hiccups. Hiccups began while I was at work, the day following my first treatment. That was awkward. By the time I got home, they were intense. My condition only got worse, and Gwen finally called the doctor at 8:00 p.m. These were not just simple hiccups. They were jolting! He prescribed a medication that would stop the flexing of my diaphragm that was causing the hiccups. Gwen rushed to the pharmacy. By the time she got there, it was after the closing time of 9:00 p.m., but the pharmacist waited for her. I was able to sleep that night, only because of that drug. Without it, the hiccups were too disruptive for me to rest. That reaction occurred several times following the injections.

The worst part of the treatments started as I entered the doctor's office for my fifth treatment. The moment that I walked into the doctor's office, I became very nauseated. The smell of the doctor's office made me ill. My difficulties escalated with each treatment. Nearing the day of my last treatment, I became nauseated thinking about it, even before I got to the doctor's office. That smell was so real in my mind that I dreaded entering the building. By the time that I walked into the doctor's office, it was a serious struggle to put up with that odor. I knew that it was a mental game at that point, but it was very difficult to overcome.

In December 1993, I had concluded my eight treatments and was required to take another CT scan. The purpose of this CT scan was to determine if my cancer was gone. Once again, we had to wait on the test results. Physical examinations by the oncologist appeared to show that the size of the lymph nodes was reduced by the treatments, but the conclusive evidence was in the results of the CT scans. We had to wait four days for the results. Time seemed to almost stand still. It is always that way when you are anxiously awaiting anything. Finally, I received the call from the oncologist's office. The scan results showed that my lymph nodes were near normal size again. Scarring of the nodes kept the nodes from returning to a completely normal size. My cancer was in remission. That was such great news for me, for my family and our friends. Our prayers had been answered. The oncologist made an interesting comment to me during the visit in which he ordered the CT scans. As he concluded our meeting, he said, "You have a higher chance of dying from a car accident than dying from this lymphoma. You should have a long life. I would not worry about the cancer beating you." Those comments have always stuck in my mind. He assured me that the cancer would return, but to him it was obvious that my body was responding to the chemotherapy in a very positive way. It was apparent that he believed what he was saying. It was not just a comment to make me feel better. That comment provided me with a lot of strength to face the cancer in the future. It made me feel more confident to hear him express his confidence that I would be successful in my fight.

About two months after treatment, my hair began growing again. Something totally unexpected occurred. My new hair was darker than it was prior to any treatments, and it was very wavy in the back. In the past, I did not like my hair to curl, but the new, wavy hair was just fine with me. My hair was thicker than before I lost it, so why be concerned. I was just glad to have hair again! By April 1994, I had a full head of hair. I was feeling great. I had my first checkup following the treatments in March. All of my blood workup revealed very positive numbers. I was starting to lose the weight that I had gained as a result of the Prednizone. Everything was positive in my life again. I was so grateful that my cancer was in remission.

My brother invited Gwen and me to join him and his wife on a weekend trip to La Jolla, CA, shortly after I received the great news. Gwen and I were excited to get away. We arrived late Friday afternoon and found our hotel. After we took our luggage to our room, we realized that we still had time to walk along the beach before sunset. We took a quick stroll on the beach. Going through all of the stress and anxiety associated with a potentially terminal illness, causes you to appreciate so many things that you once took for granted. When we were walking the beach at La Jolla, the smallest things meant so much more to me. The depth of appreciation that I should have always felt was finally there. Unfortunately, we seldom know how great something is until it is taken from us, or we lose it. My gratitude for each additional day of life that I have is now realized. Before, "tomorrow" was something that I just expected to happen. It is a great change when we start to realize how precious life is. We all should have that kind of thankfulness and gratitude for the small things in life, as well as the great gifts.

That evening, we were able to have dinner with my nieces. On Saturday, all of us were together and had a great day. We had a little time to kill on Sunday afternoon, so Gwen and I drove around town. Driving along the shoreline, we found a small park and an area where seals were relaxing on the rocks. It was an overcast day, so I cannot call it "basking in the sun", but they were being very lazy and enjoying the small audience. We parked our car and walked over to the cliff, which was about twenty feet higher than where the seals were lying. Then Gwen decided that she wanted to take a picture of me near the cliff. There was a two-inch pipe railing outlining the edge of the cliff. I walked over to the pipe railing and turned to pose for the picture. As I posed, I leaned back against the railing. When Gwen looked into the camera viewfinder, she did not see me. Then she looked up and found me lying on the ground, on top of the fence railing, right at the edge of the cliff. I was within inches of falling over the cliff into very jagged rocks.

Gwen came running over to see if I was okay. She quickly knew that I was fine. I was laying there laughing and thinking, "What else? I just went through chemotherapy and have survived cancer, only to kill myself while having my picture taken? That figures!" Once Gwen realized that I was fine, we both started laughing and joking about the way our luck was going. We started examining the railing and noticed that the pipe was nearly rusted through at all of the welded joints. Apparently, that railing had been there for an extended time and the seawater had been eating at it. At the time, I thought I needed to contact the city government and inform them of a potentially dangerous situation. Unfortunately, that thought soon passed and I never called, like I should have done. The remainder of our weekend was very enjoyable and we hated that it had to end.

For the next three years, I had a check-up visit with the oncologist every three months and a CT scan every six months. I always had that anxious period of three to five days, waiting on the test results following the scans. I was in good health, but I knew the possibility was always there that the test results would reveal that the cancer had returned. The oncologist had told me from the beginning that I would suffer multiple occurrences of the non-Hodgkins lymphoma. There was, and still is no cure for it.

Chapter 2

Recurring Cancer

In June 1997, I was lying in bed one night, and I began feeling around on my body, searching for any enlarged nodes. Doing that had become a common practice for me. I would examine my neck; under my chin; under my armpits; and my groin. Lymph nodes lie near the skin in each of those areas, so it is easy to find an inflamed node. I found enlarged lymph nodes on the right side of my neck. My heart sank when I felt the nodules. I knew that my cancer had returned. I prayed to God that it was not cancer, or if it was, that the treatments would be successful once again. Gwen was away visiting her family at the time. When she returned, I informed her of the bad news. It appeared that the news was harder for Gwen than it was for me. She believed that I had beaten the cancer, regardless of what the doctor had told us.

We had dreaded the day that my cancer would return. That day had arrived. I had been in remission for almost four years to the day. I was looking forward to five years, but it did not happen. Cancer patients often talk about looking forward to being in remission for five years, because the health insurance companies typically consider you free of disease at that point. Four years was a nice, extended time to be in remission. It gave us hope that my cancer was actually cured. The news of its return was disappointing, but Gwen and I were optimistic about my prognosis. My oncologist had told us that the cancer would return, because it is not curable, but we had still hoped that my situation would be unique. After all, my battle with cancer had had numerous unique or unusual twists to it, but that was not to be one of them.

On Friday, June 13, yes, that is correct—Friday the Thirteenth, I had surgery to biopsy the enlarged nodes. I have never been a superstitious person. In fact, I like to do things on which superstitions are based just to prove them wrong. Biopsy tests of the removed lymph nodes concluded that my cancer had definitely returned. Now you might think that I should have been a little cautious about superstitions, but that had nothing to do with the positive test results. I had already found the enlarged nodes on my neck and knew what I would be facing. The confirming results were very disappointing, because you always hope that your gut feelings are wrong. There was a positive conclusion from the pathology report. The aggressive cancer had not returned. Only the low-grade lymphoma was present. CT scans were ordered again to determine the extent of the disease. Where was it this time? How much cancer existed? The news was much better. This time the cancer was only found in my neck. It was classified as Stage I disease. The extent of the disease was much less. All of that news was a true blessing. I had cancer again, but it could have been much worse. It was localized in one area, so we had definitely found it at a very early stage. Since the aggressive cancer was not present, my treatment was a little different. It was referred to as COP, which consisted of Cyclophosphamide, Vincristine (Oncovintin) and Prednizone. That was more good news! My body did not have to be subjected to the drug, Adriamiacin, which can cause heart damage.

Six chemotherapy treatments were prescribed for my second cancer occurrence. The first three treatments were administered with no side effects. The appointments were scheduled for 4:00 on Thursday afternoons so I only missed about two hours of work. After the appointment, I went home and relaxed for the remainder of the evening. I was only able to eat a very lite meal, such as soup and crackers. On Friday morning, I was back at work, ready to go. I even played basketball at lunchtime on Friday afternoons. The group that I played basketball with showed up every Monday, Wednesday and Friday at noon to play. Playing basketball was very therapeutic for me. It provided a tremendous diversion from the current stresses, plus it got the competitive juices flowing. For that hour to hour and a half, I could forget about everything but the game at hand. Following a treatment, my body was lethargic as I played, but I pushed myself to exercise as much as possible. About seven days after each treatment, my legs felt like jelly. I could not jump. I was used to shooting jump shots, but my legs had no spring. That was a very minor setback. I was more than willing to live with that little problem. All the guys that played basketball were amazed that I was able to play while I was receiving chemotherapy. Their support was greatly appreciated. When I asked the oncologist about exercise, he had told me to do whatever I felt like doing, so I did. The big difference between my first chemotherapy treatments and this series was that I was not required to take the Adriamiacin. If it had been required, I would not have been able to exercise as vigorously as I did.

After the fourth, fifth and sixth treatments, I ran a low-grade fever on Thursday night and Friday following each treatment, plus my stomach was very unsettled. That caused me to miss a total of three days of work, but I did have a laptop that allowed me to work from home. On Fridays, I would dial into the office, check my e-mail and respond as necessary. If I had some documents to write, I would work on them. I just did not feel well enough to go to work on those Fridays following treatment. By Saturday, I felt normal again. Because I was taking Prednizone, I had all of the same symptoms as I did during my first chemotherapy treatments. While taking

Prednizone, it was like I was taking "uppers." I was "zooming"; did not require much sleep, nor was I able to sleep. I was wide-awake and ready to do things. That nervous energy and anxiety soon left after I stopped taking the steroid. In addition, I did not lose as much hair during the second round of treatments, primarily because I was not taking the Adriamiacin. Unfortunately, my remission only lasted for twenty-one months this time. It appeared that my body had built up immunities to the chemotherapy drugs, and they were not as effective the second time.

During the time that I was receiving treatments, Gwen and I made every effort to minimize the negative impact on our children. Balancing our daily lives between doctor's visits, work, summer sports and school activities was a real challenge. There were days that I did not go to work, which was not the norm for me, so it was obvious that something was different. Our small town rallied around our children and many families became an extension of our family. Gwen's outward appearance was very strong. She did not appear to be phased by the reality of more treatments and insecurity. But, she later told me that she shed many tears while in the shower. That was a secret place for her, where no one could hear her sobbing, or feel her pain.

Today, many of our friends are amazed at how "mentally strong" Gwen and I appear to be. We have learned to deal with adversity quite well. Our friends know what all has gone on in our lives since my cancer was discovered for the first time in 1993 and cannot believe how we continue to live a full, happy life. The return of my cancer in June 1997 was the first of several life-changing events that my family faced over a five-year period. Many of our friends were shocked that all of those bad situations could happen to one family. Friends would make comments to us like, "I can't believe that all of this is happening to you"; or, "I don't know how you all do it"; or, "When is this all going to end for you all?" The chapters that follow will elaborate on those life-altering situations, thus I will only briefly identify those events to which I am referring for now.

June 1997—CT scans revealed that my cancer had returned after four years in remission. I had six chemo treatments from July to December.

October 17, 1998—Our house was flooded with seventeen feet of water; lost all of our furniture and most of our clothing, plus I lost approximately $60,000 worth of sports memorabilia; had no flood insurance, but four months later found out we should have had it; and because of persistence and months of written communication with the mortgage company, they paid to have the house rebuilt

December 1998—CT scans confirmed that my non-Hodgkin's lymphoma had returned after 21 months of remission—received twenty radiation treatments on left side of neck

June 27, 1999—My brother, my only sibling, died at the age of fifty-one of heat stroke while hiking

July 2000—CT scans confirmed my cancer had returned — received twenty radiation treatments on right side of neck

November 11, 2000—Gwen's mother died of complications from diabetes and congestive heart failure after a two-year health battle. She was one of my strongest supporters. We had a very solid relationship.

December 2000—CT scans confirmed my cancer had returned at stage III, meaning above and below diaphragm; started treatment of Rituxan, a new drug introduced November, 1997; still in remission as of this writing

June 21, 2002—My mother had a massive stroke; she had brain surgery to remove a tennis ball sized blood clot; her right side was paralyzed, blind in the right eye and only had about five percent of her vocabulary, because of the location of the clot and the related brain damage.

August 31, 2002—My father committed suicide; he could not stand to see my mother in pain and was frustrated because she could not talk much; he finally realized that she would never return home

November 3, 2002—My mother died while under the loving care of Hospice

Several unique situations occurred following my third recurrence of cancer in 1998. Enlarged lymph nodes were found under my right jawbone, and one just below my neck in the chest. For the third time, surgery was performed to confirm that the nodules were malignant. The surgeon removed the nodule under my jawbone. This time, the oncologist's approach was different. My oncologist expressed a great deal of concern about the health and strength of my immune system. He emphasized the need to consider various treatment alternatives since I had already been through two different series of chemotherapy. The density of the white blood count in my bone marrow was lessened with each series of chemotherapy treatments, thus my immune system's effectiveness was weakened. When the oncologist warned me of the potential damage to my immune system, it was obvious that we had to proceed with caution. My oncologist suggested that I consider a stem cell harvest for a possible bone marrow transplant. He recommended me to another oncologist, who specialized in clinical trials on bone marrow transplants. This option was somewhat appealing, because the research was conducted at the University Hospital in San Antonio, Texas. I felt very fortunate that I only lived about forty-five miles away from one of the leading research centers for bone marrow transplants. At the same time, the idea of a bone marrow transplant seemed extreme. I felt great. I was playing basketball regularly. How could I need something that drastic?

It was amazing when we met with the research oncologist during our first consultation. She was a young, neat person; someone who did not seem old enough to have much research experience, but she certainly did. Her mannerisms were very calming. As she discussed my situation and elaborated on her past experience, I became very confident in her expertise. She explained that the only options for a bone marrow transplant (within their trials) were using bone marrow from a sibling or from me. That led to several different tests. My brother was tested to see if he was a match to be a bone marrow donor. He was not a match and he was my only sibling, so the only remaining option was an autologous sample, meaning that stem cells from my bone marrow would be harvested for a future transplant. In order for my bone marrow to be acceptable, tests had to be run to show that my bone marrow was free from any cancer. Step one was to extract a bone marrow sample. The oncologist had performed numerous extractions of bone marrow samples from various patients. Manual drilling was required and she had to exert an extreme amount of pressure to break through to the cavity of the bone.

I was lying flat on my stomach as she exerted downward pressure and twisted the drilling syringe. The sample was taken from the pelvis bone in the small of the back. Oddly enough, there was not any real pain. It was just the sensation of constant pressure being applied to my lower back. Of course, by natural tendency was to stiffen my back to counteract the pressure, but that was the wrong thing to do. Several minutes into the procedure, it was obvious that my bone density was so thick that she could hardly drill through my pelvis. Gwen was in the examination room at the time, observing the doctor drilling into my pelvis. She could hardly stand to watch, because the doctor had to work so hard physically to break through the bone. Gwen also stated that she would never be in the room again when that procedure had to be performed. The bone itself does not contain nerve endings, so the drilling did not bother me until the drill reached the bone marrow cavity about thirty minutes into the process, which was much longer than anticipated. As the drill broke into the marrow cavity, the pain was like a strong toothache. It was deep and aching, but it was tolerable. It is not possible to deaden the cavity of the bone. Finally, a sample was extracted and sent to the lab to determine if cancer was present in bone marrow. A few days later, the oncologist called me while I was at work. She informed me that she had received the test results from my bone marrow and that she had good news and bad news. My response was, "Why should anything be different now? Nothing is ever typical with my cancer. Why change now?" She laughed with me; then proceeded to explain the situation. According to microscopic viewing of the sample, no presence of cancer was detected. Great news, however, the conclusive factor in determining the presence of cancer required that my blood contained a specific cell type, a Bcl-2 cell type. Seventy-five percent of all patients have this Bcl-2 cell type, but I did not. Now a decision had to be made as to whether, or not, we would go through with the process of an aphaeresis to harvest stem cells for a potential bone marrow transplant in the future, knowing that there was a possibility that my bone marrow contained cancer. There was some real anxiety in weighing the alternatives. Of course, there was disappointment in the fact that my body did not contain the Bcl-2 cell type, but I kept reminding myself "things could be a lot worse." At least I was alive and had options to consider. In the end the choice was mine to make. Gwen was willing to support me in whatever decision I made. Certainly, the doctor left the final decision to me, because there was no "wrong" answer. My initial reaction was that I did not have much of a choice, but I called Gwen to discuss the alternatives prior to confirming my decision with the doctor. Gwen agreed that I should proceed with the stem cell harvest. Capturing stem cells from my body was the only real option available to me. We were fairly certain that the marrow was clear. I chose to do the aphaeresis. Prior to the harvest, my body had to be stimulated to generate huge amounts of stem cells. That is a standard procedure. The doctor prescribed the vials of medication, which I had to receive via injections for four consecutive days. This was definitely one time when having a prescription card, as part of my health insurance was a true blessing. We had to call the pharmacy and ask them to order the required dosage, because they did not inventory that drug. When we went to the pharmacy to pick up the special order vials, the pharmacist commented that they were very expensive. We asked, "What do you mean by that?" She stated that each vial pack was $4,800. Thanks to the prescription card, I only had to pay the $15 out-of-pocket co-pay. My next decision was whether I would drive 45 miles to the hospital twice a day for a thirty second injection, or find someone in New Braunfels to give me the injections. Fortunately, we had a very close friend who was a nurse. She was more than happy to administer the eight daily injections that were required—four in the morning and four in the evening, over a four-day period. That was a huge savings of time and wear-and-tear on the car. Now it was time for the actual stem cell harvest. The medical term for the process is an aphaeresis. Very few hospitals are equipped for this procedure. The doctor prepared me for the aphaeresis by explaining that it would require being connected to the machine two to three days, four hours at a time, to collect the needed number of stem cells. The aphaeresis process is very similar to dialysis, so I was told. To prepare for the procedure, the first step was to have a shunt inserted in my upper chest area. This would provide for easy connectivity to the "stem cell strainer" machine, to put it in terms I can understand. The shunt was inserted and I was taken to the room where I was connected. In a period of about four hours, all of my blood was cycled out of my body, into the machine where stem cells were collected, then the blood was reinserted into my body. As the blood was returned to my body, it was combined with a citrus concentrate, which kept the blood from coagulating.

The goal was to harvest two million stem cells. After I completed the first aphaeresis appointment, they told me that they would submit the harvested stem cells for a count, then call me in the afternoon to schedule the next appointment. I had already scheduled the next day off from work. When the call came that afternoon, everyone was totally blown away (surprised)! A total of six million cells had been harvested the first day and there was no need for me to go through the process a second time. That was great news, but atypical. Why should anything be normal?

The final task was for me to return to the hospital so the shunt could be removed. The nursing staff said that it was a very simple procedure to remove the shunt from my chest. According to their estimates, I would only be there for 30 minutes to an hour. It did not turn out to be quite that simple. Why should it? Nothing else had been. I told Gwen that she could go to work the next day. It was my opinion that there was no need for her to miss anymore work and ride with me to the hospital. She was not convinced, but went along with my request. I arrived at the hospital and they were quick to accommodate me. I was positioned on the same table where the shunt had been inserted. When the nurse pulled the tube from my chest, an excruciating pain in my chest overcame me. I could not breathe and it burned so badly that it was unbearable. Have you ever swallowed a pill, only for it to go down sideways? That really hurts, but this pain was at least fifty times worse. I thought that I was suffering a heart attack. The nurse asked me to explain what was wrong. It was difficult to speak, but she got the message. She had never experienced this kind of reaction before. She had removed patients' shunts many, many times before. She called for immediate assistance. After about ten minutes, the pain subsided, and I was moved to a patient's room for an extended observation period. Nurses speculated that there were small traces of the citrus concentrate lingering in the tube that dripped out while the tube was being extracted, and that caused the severe pain. This was a specialty hospital that specialized in bone marrow transplant research. Aphaeresis procedures were conducted on a routine basis at this hospital, but only one nurse had ever seen this kind of reaction. And she had only seen this happen one or two times in the many years that she had been doing this. Everything about the stem cell harvest process was unique.

Finally, about 1:30 p.m., I stopped by Gwen's office after my hospital visit. Based on what the hospital staff had told me, I expected to be home by 11:00, but that was assuming that everything went as planned. When I showed up in her office, Gwen was worrying about me. I laughed about the situation and told her that it did not go quite as smoothly as they said it would. She then thought about what all could have gone wrong and the fact that she was not there. At that point, she made it clear to me that she would never again let me go alone for any hospital procedure, other than my regular CT scans.

Today, we joke saying "if something is going to be unusual or atypical, then it is going to happen to me." That is just the way that every phase of my cancer experience has been from the initial diagnosis; to the first pathology report; to the aphaeresis; to my current remission with the drug Rituxan.

"Unusual" as in my initial diagnosis and subsequent surgery results. Both my family doctor and my surgeon felt certain that my surgery would be very minor, and would be for nothing more than to remove a thyroid cyst. Lymph nodes are typically not found just below your chin. They are more likely on the side of your neck. It was my first surgery ever, but I was not very nervous, because I was going to have surgery, be back home in two hours and back to work in nine days. Nine days may sound like a long time, but the surgeon speculated that the cyst would be close to my larynx, thus requiring a deep incision and an extended recovery period. No big deal, I thought. The doctors had assured me that the "cyst" was nothing to worry about. Based on my then clean medical history, I felt that they were probably right. In the end, it was cancer, not a benign cyst. And, I could have been back to work the following Monday from a physical recovery perspective—not the nine days estimated before the surgery. Bad news.

"Atypical" as in my first pathology report contrasted to my second reading. First, my surgeon informed me that the pathology report indicated that I had Hodgkin's disease! That blew me away! But we thought that was better than non-Hodgkin's lymphoma, based on our research. We thought we had received the best news of the two possibilities, only to be told on our first visit with the oncologist that I did in fact have non-Hodgkin's lymphoma. Not the best news.

The fact that my blood cells did not contain the cancer marker that 75% of people have was atypical. There was no way to verify that my bone marrow did not contain cancer.

The results of my aphaeresis were very much atypical. The doctor had assured me that I would have to spend at least two days connected to the machine in order to harvest enough stem cells. In one day, they were able to harvest three times as many cells as hoped for. Great news!

Removing the port from my chest after the aphaeresis was complete and what happened was "unusual." The pain that I suffered was excruciating. I just knew that I was having a heart attack. Then, I could tell by the look on the nurse's face and her actions that my reactions were totally unexpected. Of all the nurses that saw me in the next hour, only one nurse could recall just one other patient that had ever experienced the same pain from the removal of the port. Scary news.

The length of my remission following my treatments with Rituxan was "atypical." The doctor told me that I would be in remission for nine to fifteen months. He assured me that I would need more treatments. As of this writing, I have been in remission 56 months. Awesome news! I like being atypical when it means fewer treatments and a healthier life!

Chapter 3

You Are Not the Only One Impacted by Your Cancer

My point in sharing the treatment experience is to express that I did have some difficult times during treatment, but I realized how important it was to continue the treatments. I saw fellow patients that just gave up on the treatments, because of the sickening side effects. My wife spoke to some of their family, and their family members were discouraged by the decision that the patient had made to stop treatments. That decision impacts more than just the patient. It has a tremendous impact on friends and family that love the patient. Friends and family lose hope when the patient gives up. As a patient, do you want to add that burden to your loved ones? It is one thing for them to know that you did everything that the doctor recommended; yet it did not work and in the end you passed away. It is another thing for you to give up on the treatments; stop going, and they never know what the outcome would have been, had you followed through with everything the doctor recommended. I have also known of several people who took the treatments for a long time and did not see the results that they desired and they, along with their family members, jointly decided to stop the treatments. If you want to stop the treatments, I believe that it would be best to first discuss that choice with those near and dear to you during the treatment process. The ultimate decision can only be made by the patient. Family members then need to accept the patient's decision.

It is very important that you openly discuss your disease with your immediate family. I did not realize just how great an impact that my cancer had on my children until they were completely stressed out at times and then one of them would mention their concern about the effects of my cancer on me as one of their major concerns. One of my sons "went off" one day. As he later talked about what led up to that, he stated, "school sucks; our football season is horrible; Dad was diagnosed with cancer again, and…" Until that time, he never voiced his concern to me. And, yes, I know that it had to bother him, but he never indicated in anyway how much it concerned him. We would openly discuss the cancer, and he appeared to be okay with it. If you have a good relationship with your children, then you receive a bad health diagnosis, understand that your children will be impacted by that uncertainty entering their lives. Realize that each child will deal with the situation in his or her own way. Their security is shaken. They may be thinking that they could lose one of their parents. Their next thought may be, "Would that mean that they would also be losing their home?" or, "How would things change?" Your children will have questions like these running through their head, but they may never voice them. You need to look for changes in their routines. Are they all of a sudden withdrawing from you? Or, withdrawing from their friends? Do they seem depressed? Are they gone from home more, avoiding the situation? How are their grades—are they dropping? Has their behavior at school changed?

It is not easy to assess the impact that the diagnosis of cancer, or some other major illness, will have on your children, particularly in their teenage years. My two oldest children are boys. As teenagers, they were never willing to openly express their feelings on any emotion related topic.

They only seemed to be open about something that they wanted very badly. Young children tend to be more expressive of their feelings when asked, mostly due to their innocence, I believe. That is not the case with teenage children. You need to pay special attention to their actions in order to gain an understanding. You may need to ask leading questions that will cause them to express their feelings without them realizing that they are doing so. If you have a good relationship with some of their best friends, look for opportunities to speak to their friends in private. You may not want your children to know that you are approaching their friends. It is important to let the friends know that you are just trying to understand the situation. Assure the friends that your children will not be in trouble for anything that they bring up. Once the friends understand that you value their insight, they can become a very valuable resource to you in understanding your children.

In many aspects, the impact on my children has been very positive. They have learned the cold, hard lesson that we have no guarantee that our lives will remain as we plan them to be. It has made them stronger, because they recognize that life is not always pleasant. They recognize that each of us will be faced with challenges and the important thing to keep in mind is to remain positive at all times. Understanding that trying times are just part of life helps them to cope with change. That is not to say that it makes difficult times easy, but it does keep them from being so traumatic.

When I am right in the middle of the battle with the disease, I do not necessarily realize the impact that it has on others. The effect it has on others is manifested in different ways to different people. In 1993, after my first diagnosis, I was going through chemotherapy and my mother-in-law came to Texas from Oklahoma to visit. She was visiting for the first time since our move. Gwen had told her how well I was doing with the treatments. I was doing great! I felt good, but my mother-in-law had not seen me in nine months. The last time she saw me, I was a "picture of health." I had a full head of hair. I was fit, having just returned from a week at the Mickey Mantle / Whitey Ford fantasy camp. When my mother-in-law arrived at our house, she came into the living room, gave me a big hug and she seemed fine, but then she went into the kitchen pantry, shut the door and began to sob. Later she told Gwen that she was not prepared for how I looked. I had no hair and my face was round. I was twenty pounds over weight due to the Prednizone that was part of my chemotherapy and my skin tones were grayish. I had received a treatment that day and I had dark circles around my eyes. If you have been through chemotherapy treatments, or experienced someone going through them, you know the look that I am describing. To Gwen and me, I was doing great. We had grown accustomed to the changes in my physical appearance. To my mother-in-law who had not seen me since my diagnosis of cancer, I looked like a ghost with a heartbeat.

My diagnosis of cancer changed my life in a very positive way. I was a vain person before cancer. Friends at church would comment about how my hair was always perfect, with no hairs ever out of place. I would blow-dry my hair every morning just so that it would not curl on the ends or have waves. I would get a haircut when Gwen did not think I needed one, but I wanted my hair to look good. As I mentioned earlier, two weeks after my first chemotherapy treatment, my hair started falling out in globs. My outlook on my physical appearance totally changed. I did not care any more. I was just appreciating the fact that I was alive and that my cancer had been diagnosed before it was too far along.

We openly joked about the way I looked. Some of my friends gave me a funny baseball cap with an attached ponytail. When I wore it, it looked like I had a ponytail sticking out the back, but on the front it read, "Having a bad hair day." According to my kids, the round face, dark circles around my eyes and bald head made me a perfect candidate for an "Uncle Fester" photo. A sense of humor will get you through a lot of tough situations. It is also important to let your friends know that you are comfortable with them joking about your recently bald head. That will help everyone cope better while being around you. Many people were very uncomfortable when they first saw me after I was diagnosed with cancer, and then again when my hair fell out. They did not know what to say—what could they say that would not make me feel bad, or thought, "Is it okay to discuss it?" It was hard for others to mention the "C" word around me. I tried to make it clear to my friends that I was okay with hearing and saying, "I have cancer." I often tell friends, "I don't get sick. I just get cancer." That will usually generate some laughter, and, at the same time, it is a highly accurate statement.

In addition to my hair loss, my face was disfigured because of the Prednizone. One of the side effects of Prednizone is the changing of your facial features like an enlarged, protruding forehead. Additionally, Prednizone caused me to gain thirty-five pounds during treatment. A lot of people lose weight while on chemotherapy treatments, but not me. I put on thirty-five pounds and ballooned to the largest weight of my life, about 250 pounds. At 6'2", I looked like a bouncer in a club with my shaved head and big body. Being overweight was out of the norm for me. I had always prided myself for staying in good physical condition. That is the pride in me that is not necessarily a good trait. The importance that I placed on my physical appearance changed. This kind of physical change in appearance was something that would have embarrassed me in times past. But, knowing that I was battling cancer, I did not worry about those things. Plus, it was not good for me to worry. It was much more important for me to concentrate on the positive aspects of my body being treated and responding positively to those treatments. If and when I regained my health, I knew that I would work to get rid of that extra weight. When the hair started to return, it was surprising. My hair had a lot of gray in it before the cancer, but it grew back much darker. In addition, a lot of my hair was very curly, and you know what? I did not care any more. I was just glad to have hair again. I did not use the blow dryer again for years.

In recent times, I have been humbled by comments made by some of my superiors at work. During a training session, my boss made the following comments. "Gene continues to be such an inspiration to me. I am amazed at all the things that he and his family have been through, and how he is always so bright and cheerful. You would never know that he was dealing with problems." Another executive has introduced me to others and expressed how great an example I have been for him in the way that I have faced and dealt with adversity. These are individuals that I never consciously worked to impress with my smile and approach to life. It was very touching for me to hear their comments about their admiration for me. Again, you never know who is watching you, or whose life you will impact.

Chapter 4

Coincidence?

Based on circumstances that surrounded my first three recurrences of cancer, I just knew that in my situation, there had to be a direct link between the cancer and the physical trauma and stress that my body was subjected to prior to each recurrence. With multiple recurrences, I have tried to determine if there were any issues, causes or unusual stress present prior to each instance that the disease started. This is what I discovered.

Cancer appeared for the first time following my broken wrist that occurred during my participation in a Mantle-Ford Fantasy baseball camp. The accident occurred in November 1992 and it was my first broken bone ever. I leaped, outstretched for a low line drive. The end of my glove stuck in the grass, causing my glove and hand to fold underneath my arm. Seven months later, in June 1993, I was diagnosed with cancer. At that point, there was no reason to think that my broken arm had anything to do with my cancer. As already detailed, in December 1993, after six months of treatments, I was declared in remission. Then, in 1997, four years after my first treatments, I was playing in a league basketball game. While running the court on a fast break, I collided with a spectator who was walking out on the court at the wrong time. I tried to catch my fall with my left hand and broke two fingers. Six weeks later, my cancer returned. Prior to breaking my fingers, there was no indication of cancer, so that made me think that there might be a correlation between my body being subjected to trauma and my cancer being reactivated. When I was initially diagnosed, the doctor showed me where the lumps would be most obvious, and how to identify them in the future. From that point on, I have examined myself for tumors on a regular basis. That is the reason I stated that there was no evidence that there was any cancer in my body. Now, at the same time, I could not feel my cancer in every spot.

When I met with the doctor after my second diagnosis, I discussed my theory with him. I explained to him the events that took place prior to each diagnosis. To me, it was more than just coincidence, but my doctor was certain that it was only a matter of coincidence. Even after that conversation, I was still convinced that there was a direct link between the broken bones and the cancer.

With the third recurrence, the situation was a little different, but it was still physical stress. In October 1998, my life was suddenly filled with stress when our house was flooded. When I say flooded, I'm talking about seventeen feet of water. We had three feet of water in our second story. Literally, a river was running through our house at the time. Our whole community was declared a national disaster area. The stress stemmed from the fact that we did not have any flood insurance, so the mental and emotional stress was enormous. There will be more on the flood later. In December 1998, my cancer reoccurred for the third time. Thus, I felt that there had to be a definite connection between the trauma, whether physical or emotional, and my cancer continuing to reoccur.

However, in the spring of 2001, I was playing basketball and my face collided with another player's shoulder (if you get what I mean), breaking my nose. Surgery was required and I could not play basketball for two months. It was a very significant break, with my nose pushed off to one side. Prior to the surgery it was so obvious that my nose was broken, because of how crooked it was. My cancer has not reappeared since that accident, so that blew my theory, thank goodness.

The point is, you may have similar thoughts. You may search to identify anything that you can do, or quit doing, to stop the cancer from returning. In my particular case, my theory was wrong, but it took a long time for me to believe that. My oncologist was correct, but I was not immediately convinced that he was. You should educate yourself about your condition, question recommendations, and take ownership of your health. In my mind, it is okay to have your own theories, but do not discredit everything that your doctor says. Value their knowledge, and compare it with the knowledge you have gained through your research. Ultimately, you should choose what is best for you, and stand by your decision, regardless of how popular it is with your doctor. Hopefully, you will have an oncologist, with whom you can freely share your thoughts. If you do not, then it may be time to search for one who will listen to your input. You know your body better than anyone. You know how you normally feel, and you know when something is not right. What is normal for one person will not necessarily be normal for you. With new information that I have been studying, I am convinced that nutritional supplements must be an integral part of my fight against cancer. Many professionals that practice traditional medicine do not understand the value of optimal nutrition. I have to take the matter into my own hands.

Chapter 5

Things Could Be Much Worse!

"It could be a lot worse!" Even though I usually say it as a joking reply, that phrase means a great deal to me. Oftentimes around the office, someone will ask, "How are things goin'?", or "How ya doin'?" On days when everything seems to be going wrong, I reply, "Oh, things could be a lot worse!" Sometimes, I just say it for attention. Yes, I finally admitted it! I need attention like everyone else. It is a phrase I use a lot, but it has a very important message. The phrase causes some people to stop and think, and that is my targeted response.

No matter how bad things may seem, just stop and look around for a minute. How many friends do you have? How many little luxuries do you have—Color TV or maybe a flat screen TV? New laptop computer? Maybe a new car? You could be living in Uganda, Iraq or Haiti where there is a great deal of poverty and uncertainty. Do you have AIDS? If the answer to that last question is NO, then things could be a whole lot worse! AIDS is such a horrifying disease. Consider all the people and things around you. Count the number of material things you have. Do you have any loving, caring friends? Having a great friend that you "lean on" at times and confide in is a true blessing. Having several close friends is even better. One of my favorite religious songs is "Count Your Blessings." It starts, "When upon life's billows you are tempest tossed; when you are discouraged thinking all is lost, count your many blessings—name them one by one, and it will surprise you what the Lord hath done." That is so true, but it is not easy to focus on the positive side when life seems so bad that you want it all to end. If you ever get to that point, try to recall just how blessed you really are. I know that it is a lot easier to say what to do when you are not faced with that situation, but I have been faced with those situations. It is possible for you to focus on all of the positive things that you have in your life. And, it will help you if you can! Too many times we forget just how good we have it!

On June 20, 1993, the phrase "things could be a lot worse" took on a whole new meaning for me. That was the day that my surgeon confirmed that I had cancer. Gwen and I did what we had to do—we put on a good "front." Right!? We were both thinking, "I have to be strong for him (her)." As we left the room, the surgeon had us go to an area where his receptionist would join us and provide us with contact information for an oncologist. We waited for a few minutes. I looked at Gwen and she started crying, then tears came to my eyes. We could not hold back any longer. The news was official. The pathology report confirmed the doctor's concern immediately following the surgery. Could things really be any worse? At that time, it did not seem possible. Sure they could have been, but we did not think about that then. In our minds "What could be worse?" I was the only person providing an income for the family at the time. Gwen had not been in the workforce for several years, because the kids were young—ages eight, ten and twelve. Our sense of security dropped to an all time low.

When we left the doctor's office, we had twenty minutes before we had to meet the rest of Garrett's All-star baseball team. He had a game that afternoon, and we were going to caravan to the baseball game. We drove away from the surgeon's office, and while on the way to pick up Garrett, I was approaching the hotel where I had lived for two months while I was commuting from Tulsa to New Braunfels a few months earlier. That hotel was my "home away from home." I pulled into the parking lot; drove to the back of the property; parked, and we had a good cry while holding one another. We knew we had to get all of the emotional feelings out of our system. In about five minutes we had to pick up our son and act like everything was just great. We sure did not want him worrying about my bad news before his first all-star game. At one point, Gwen began to laugh. She said, "If someone were to see us back here, they would probably think that we were having an affair!"

We made it! We put on our 'game face'. We picked up Garrett, met the ball team, and headed out of town to the game. During baseball practices earlier in the week, Gwen had mentioned to one parent that we were waiting on test results. Prior to the game, we let one of the parents know that we had received the results. During that game, a parent told us, "You ought to talk to my mother-in-law, Billie." Billie was the grandmother of one of the boys on the team. She had been treated for the same type of cancer three years earlier and was in remission. Gwen sought out Billie at the game and began talking to her. I was nearby. Billie was great. Billie was full of life, very gracious and had the confidence of a champion. Gwen was captivated by Billie's story and barely paid attention to the baseball game, except when Garrett was batting. Billie made it clear that if I became depressed or ill, that she would come to our house and help Gwen. She taught us a lot about what to expect when I started chemotherapy; how there would be good days and bad days, etc. Billie was a tremendous comfort for us. We were very lucky to have a friend like her. Things could have been much worse without people like her to encourage us and share their experiences. A few years later, Billie lost her battle with cancer. My hope is that we expressed enough gratitude to her so that she understood how important and helpful she was to us.

The next two to three days were the most difficult time for me. It took that time to deal with the situation. I am a very analytical person who needs time to think about things. For me, that is time in thought that I need to be alone and consider the whole picture. As much as anything, it was the insecurity of my family's financial future that concerned me. It was hard to come to grips with the fact that I was facing a potential life-ending disease. That was something totally new for me to experience. I had always been the healthy person, who rarely felt badly. Once the word was out that I had cancer, friends came out of the woodwork to support us. The number of cards and letters I received was amazing. That support helped me overcome any depression or uncertainty.

I often reflect on the fact that I have so much with which God has blessed me. My life could be so much worse than it is. Yes, my family has dealt with several life-changing events in a relatively short period of time. However, I still have my immediate family whom I love and cherish, and who also love me. In addition, I work for a company where executives value their employees. Our company leaders encourage each employee to strive for a balanced-life, one that is not totally involved in the business. Training is provided which emphasizes the value of the family unit, the strength and support that employees receive from those relationships and we are taught principles to improve our relationships with family and co-workers. Having a loving family; working for a business that values employees and being surrounded by caring friends is true wealth, and I am blessed.

I am forever grateful that my body has responded so positively to the treatments. This has happened because God has answered my prayers. Because of that response, my life was extended until the time that new drugs were approved for treating non-Hodgkin's lymphoma, something that had not happened for over twenty years. How much more blessed could I be? If I am going to have cancer, at least it is at a time when cancer research is making huge strides towards a cure.

Treatments made me ill at times, but there was never a time when I felt sick because of the cancer. Sure, I could have been going through depression or feeling sorry for myself, but I was not. My friends and family were concerned about "how I was doing." When I said, "I am doing great", a lot of people did not believe me. They did not understand how I could have Stage III cancer and feel good at the same time. Granted, during the treatments, I did not always feel well. I did not have the energy that I normally had. I would get tired more quickly from less activity, but it was just a minor inconvenience. I had expected to feel much worse. To me, things were much better than they could have been. I was doing great.

Friends have asked, "How can you continue to be so positive?" My answer is that I feel humbled that God has allowed me to be tried by these numerous situations. To me, that shows that God believes that I have the strength to endure these trials, because he has promised us all that He will always provide a way for us to make it through any trial or temptation presented before us. My faith is strengthened greatly to think that God has the trust in me that I will endure these things. I believe that God is using my life as an example for others to see that people can survive difficult situations and they can also continue to live a peaceful, fulfilling life. What an humbling, yet soothing thought. As long as God is by my side, I have so much for which to be thankful. In Matthew 6:20, it records that Jesus said:

Matt. 6:20 But lay up for yourselves treasures in heaven, where neither moth nor rust doth corrupt, and where thieves do not break through nor steal:

When you have a treasure waiting for you, how could things be any better? Our life on earth is temporary. We should be preparing for our soul's eternal destination. If we can understand how great a gift God has for us in eternity that will help us focus on doing whatever is necessary to receive that treasure.

Chapter 6

There Are NO Guarantees in Life

You may appear to be the healthiest person in the world one minute, and have a heart attack the next moment, or be hit by a truck while driving and be killed instantly. Look at what happened on September 11, 2001. Did those 3,000+ victims think their lives were in danger that morning of September 11? Absolutely not! They thought it would be like any other day—go to work, have lunch, and be back with family in the evening. It was a beautiful, clear morning; one we all love when autumn arrives. That all changed in seconds!

We should live each moment of our life as if it is our last. That includes so many things. To me that includes:

Always keeping God first in my life;

Telling and showing my wife and children that I love them on a regular basis;

Being a good example for others; and

Recognizing need and helping others when there is a need.

If you have a "dream" or life-long ambition that you have not been able to make a reality, I strongly urge you to work towards making that a reality. My dream was meeting Mickey Mantle and playing baseball in his presence. That occurred in

November 1998 when my family sent me to the Mickey Mantle / Whitey Ford Fantasy Baseball Camp in Ft. Lauderdale, FL. Attending that camp was one the most exciting times of my life! I had been a New York Yankees baseball fan since I was five years old. I remember watching "The Game of the Week" every Sunday on the CBS network in the early 60's. At the time, CBS owned the Yankees, so the Yankees games were telecast every Sunday, or that is how I remember it. Watching those games in black-and-white is still a very vivid memory in my mind. In particular, I remember the Sunday afternoon in 1964 when Bob Gibson, with the St. Louis Cardinals, was pitching in the World Series against the Yankees. Of course, Bob Gibson was one of the finest pitchers of all time. He pitched an amazing game against some of the very best players in baseball at the time—Mickey Mantle, Roger Maris, Moose Skowron, Yogi Berra, Whitey Ford, etc. At the age of 38, I got to meet and be on the baseball field with Mickey, Whitney, Moose and Yogi. I even batted against Whitney Ford. What an amazing week in my life!

The cost of the camp was $3,750 for one week of fantasy baseball. Gwen and the kids worked hard to convince me that I should spend that kind of money for myself. Garrett said that we did not need a vacation. To him, it was more important that I went to Mickey Mantle's camp than for the family to enjoy a vacation. Garrett was only seven years old at the time. It is so touching to me today to think that my seven year old son was so giving to me. I have been a life-long Yankees fan and my family knew it. Prior to that time, I had been working two jobs and the extra money that I earned from the second job paid for the camp. That was a lot of money for us and we could have used it for so many more useful things, but I do not regret spending that money on a dream trip. We drove 1,250 miles to attend the camp. Our choices for getting there were: I could go alone and fly, or we could drive as a family and have everyone there to enjoy that once-in-a-lifetime dream trip. There was no choice. Driving was the only option. I wanted to share that experience with my family. They made it possible.

I am so glad that my family convinced me to attend the camp. All campers stayed at the same hotel. We had breakfast together each morning. Then we all gathered at the Yankees Class A stadium locker room to dress and get ready for games each day. Gwen's grandmother lived nearby, so my family stayed with her and attended the camp each day as fans. My kids were even able to sit on the golf cart with Mickey. It was a time that I will never forget. I was way out of my league when it came to the financial status of most campers attending. Most of the campers were stockbrokers, doctors or attorneys who made very good money. For me, it was a second job that barely paid for the trip. The first night that I met Mickey Mantle, he even asked me, "How can a guy from Broken Arrow, OK afford to come to this camp?" His memories of Broken Arrow were from many years earlier before the city became so large. During the week of fantasy camp, no one's financial status mattered. We were all just baseball players, playing games and visiting with some of our childhood heroes. Out of eighty-four campers, there were only two men that were younger than me. That too was an indicator to me that I was out of my league, but it was a tremendous dream-come-true. Then, seven months later when I learned that I had cancer, I was even more appreciative of the time that I was able to spend at that camp. When I was diagnosed with stage III cancer, there was a good chance that I would not have another opportunity to live out a dream.

If you have children at home, remember that they will only be at home for a very short time, probably less than twenty years. I know, to some parents that can seem like an eternity but to Gwen and me, it was not long enough. And, I think that that is the way it is for many parents. Make the most of the time you do have with your children! My wife and I always made it a priority to schedule vacations, weekend trips, etc. for the entire family, not just for her and me. My children are the joy of my life! Even though they do not live at home today, we are still very involved in their lives. We look forward to spending weekends together when time permits.

Until my children graduated from high school, our lives revolved around their activities, whether it was sports or school functions. I coached my sons in summer league baseball and winter basketball. I coached my oldest son for about eight years in baseball and six years in basketball. My younger son did not respond as well to me as a coach. I took a much lesser role with his teams. My wife and I both coached our daughter's softball, plus I assisted with her basketball team. We wanted to make the most of our time with our children. Coaching provides an opportunity for you to make a tremendous impact on young people. When I coached, there was one message that I preached over and over. That was, "Winning is just gravy. The most important thing is to give your very best every moment you compete. When the game is over, do not beat on yourself for the mistakes, as long as you can honestly say that you have tried your hardest and you gave it 110%." My two sons were their own worst critics. For years, I did the same thing to myself. When I was much younger, it would take me hours after a ballgame to get over making an error during the game. I still believe in those principles that I taught. The second part of my preaching was that "You never tell anyone how good you are. You show them." If you are a skilled athlete, people will recognize your abilities. I did not want anyone developing an arrogant attitude, if I could help it. It is such a joy for me to watch a humble, skilled athlete perform with maximum effort while being the ultimate team player. There is no one more appealing to me than a successful person that is very humble, whether they are an athlete; a student; an educator or a successful person in business. That person possesses great confidence in their abilities, but displays their abilities through their actions, and not with a lot of talk. I admire people that maintain their humility and respect for others after they become successful. I wanted to instill that philosophy in not just my children, but also others that I coached.

Gwen and I enjoyed many happy times with our children, their friends and teammates. Our house was usually full of kids who needed a ride to practice, or they did not have a way to get to the game. Kids would often spend the night with us so they could ride with us to the game the next day, while their parents worked. It was important to us that these children have the opportunity to have fun and participate in the games that they loved.

When Garrett was a freshman in high school, I coached his summer AAU basketball team. My cancer reoccurred that summer for the second time. I had surgery on Friday, June 13, then I coached one of their basketball games the following Monday. Days earlier I was playing basketball with the team during practice, then the next time they saw me, my neck was heavily bandaged and had twelve staples in it, because of the surgery to remove malignant tumors. When the players saw me in that condition, it made a real impression on them. They all wanted to know what happened to me. That is when I told them that I had cancer. They were shocked. They never imagined that someone as healthy as I was could have cancer. It is common to think that people are going to look sick if they have cancer, but that is often not the case. Once someone starts going through treatment to destroy the cancer, then they start looking and feeling sick, even if they did not when they were diagnosed. It seems like you have to get sick with treatments, so you can get better later.

Coaching can also present the opportunity for you to ruin your reputation with young people if you do not treat them with respect. Do not make that mistake! Children will give you respect if you treat them fairly and are open with them. If they can tell that you are truly trying to help make them a better player and person, you will succeed with them. They have to understand that you care about them. Even when you are being very critical of them, they will appreciate you as long as it is obvious that you are doing it with their best interest in mind. And remember, "No child or young adult is trying to make errors or mistakes when participating in a game. They are not trying to make themselves look bad." However, when mistakes are made, coaches frequently lash out at them in anger, and send the message that, "You just keep making dumb plays. Get your head out of your..." After years and years of coaching, I am convinced that very few young players are trying to look bad by making mistakes. There may be a few children that will intentionally do wrong to draw attention to themselves, but there are not many. Virtually every child wants to do well, but some just do not have the hand-eye coordination, quick reflexes, or other skills, that will allow them to be any better. Simply put, they do not have the skills necessary to be a good player, but they may be the player with the biggest "heart"—they want to do well and please everyone, but are not capable. Some young players may develop skills later in life, while others never will. But, here is the KEY. If a child is trying his or her best, you need to recognize them in a positive way for their effort. Do not ridicule them for their lack of abilities. When you do that, you scar a child and destroy their self-confidence. You have no guarantee that you will get a second chance with a player that you openly embarrass or belittle. It is important that you handle the situation the right way the first time.

If you structure your spare time around your family, you will never face any regrets, if suddenly, your health changes for the worse, or heaven forbid, you were to lose one of your children. After your children leave home, you will have plenty of time to do what you want to do. Even if you do not have time afterward, what have you lost? That does not mean that you cannot do things for yourself while your children are living at home, but it does mean that you should make your family a priority. I changed the time for exercising, because I started making family a priority. Friends of mine were playing basketball during the lunch hour. For a long time, I did not join them, because I did not want to return to work sweaty. I am a person who sweats profusely when I exercise. After playing basketball for an hour, I can wring out my t-shirt in the sink. It also takes me a considerable time to cool down after a game, but I knew that I needed the exercise. Yes, I was able to take a shower after playing, but I would still sweat for the next thirty to forty-five minutes. I finally came to the conclusion that playing at noon offered too many advantages for me to not do it. My work schedule was adjusted so that I would arrive at work one-half hour early and take a longer lunch. When I returned from lunch, I would eat at my desk as I worked through my e-mail, or read technical reports. The workouts at noon provided me with the opportunity to have fun; was a great stress reliever, and it did not take time away from my family. Yes, when I returned to work, I would still be sweating a little, but I felt better. For years I was addicted to that routine. I looked forward to that time, because of the camaraderie that was developed over the years with those friends while competing against one another on the basketball court.

My attitude towards competition drastically changed after I was diagnosed with cancer. Prior to that, I was one of the most competitive people around. I was always a true team player. I never openly criticized or blamed my teammates for a loss, but I was extremely critical of myself any time I made a mistake. After I was diagnosed with cancer, I recognized just how silly it was to become so upset about a stupid game and how I might have caused us to lose. There was no doubt that

I always played my hardest, but I still did not want to accept that mistakes do happen. The biggest change in my attitude was that I started to appreciate the opportunities that I had to play games, whether it was recreational or competitive softball, basketball, volleyball or golf. Before, I just took for granted that I was healthy and strong enough to play those games. All of a sudden, it was apparent to me that "good health" is not guaranteed, but instead, it is something that I should cherish. I learned how to laugh at my mistakes rather than always getting mad. Do not take me wrong. I have not lost my competitive drive. I still love to win, but not at the price of a bad game ruining my day or week. Instead, when I am playing games, I am open about recognizing my mistakes and I am constantly encouraging others for their effort. If I see some players getting really frustrated at themselves or others, I just make a comment like "Do not worry about it. It is just a stupid game!" That often takes the edge off a little bit.

Until the age of 51, I played full-court basketball with high school and college students, along with guys in their twenties, thirties and forties. That was over twelve years after I was initially diagnosed with cancer. After two rounds of chemo, two rounds of radiation and one round of Rituxan, I was so thankful that I was able to play basketball with friends. Playing basketball was a tremendous pleasure for me. When I could not play, because of other commitments, it was like suffering from withdrawals. I enjoyed it that much. When I saw young men who were arrogant and displayed the attitude that they were invincible, I looked for opportunities to share with them that no one is invincible. Because I was still a decent basketball player, I was able to get their attention in most cases. Other players were amazed that I played at the level I did when they realized I was over 50. They were even more amazed when they learned that I had been battling cancer for over twelve years. I was not looking for any sympathy when I shared that with them. My whole point was to help them understand that life can change when we least expect it, and we need to appreciate everything that we do have today for tomorrow may be a totally different story. I would then tell them how unexpectedly I learned of my cancer.

Another reason I share my cancer experience is that I want to give others hope in a bad situation. If someone can see me as healthy as I am today, and understand that I have been through some very serious battles with cancer, it may help them to realize that their family or friends with cancer can also win the battle. I know that my first thought when I was diagnosed was, "How long do I have to live?" For most people with whom I have discussed cancer, it always equates to death in the near future. Today, that is not always the case. A positive attitude is extremely important as you go through treatment. In addition, how you approach the next treatment, or how you react to the initial diagnosis, can determine how everyone else around you is affected. Do you want those around you to have a bad experience? I did not, so I made a conscience effort to console those people. If you are a person who needs a lot of sympathy and attention, that may not work for you. I honestly did not suffer from my cancer. I want to reiterate, there are no guarantees in life, so make the most of your time by doing those things that are the most fulfilling to you and your loved ones. Do not let pride or fear of embarrassment get in the way of expressing your feelings to those closest to you.

Chapter 7

My Outlet to Others Was Writing

Over time, I have kept several emails and notes that I wrote to family members and co-workers to update them on my health, as well as to express my love and appreciation for them. This is not something that I did before I was diagnosed with cancer. It is another example of a positive change that resulted from having cancer.

I was never good at verbally expressing my true feelings to my family. A lot of words were never said that should have been. I wanted that to change. I wanted each family member to know the love that I had for them and the joy that they brought to my life. In order to do that, I turned to notes and letters. I lost the ability to control my emotions after being diagnosed with cancer. My empathy became very strong for others. If I had tried to express my feelings face-to-face, I would have never been able to hold my composure. That was a big reason for why I turned to writing. I was crying as I wrote the notes, and trying to express them verbally would have been impossible. As the years have past, I have become better at verbally expressing my feelings, but I still have a long way to go. Here are some thoughts that I recorded the first time that my cancer reappeared.

It is Father's Day, June 15, 1997. I'm 43 years old and I had surgery on Friday, the 13th, to remove 5 lymph nodes on the right side of my neck. The cancer of 4 years ago has returned. I'm not too concerned for my own personal well-being. I've been playing basketball 2-3 days a week for the last 2 years. My stamina is pretty good for a 43 year old that has a desk job. I take some pride in that.

This is the second time around to deal with cancer. My wife seems to be handling it surprisingly well. The kids do not show their emotions so I'm not sure, but I think they are doing okay. I've asked Todd and Garrett if they were okay with this and they responded, "Yes."

I went to church with my family this morning as usual. However, it is always tough for me to receive sympathy and well wishing from others. I give people the wrong impression because tears come to my eyes when someone says something nice. Mrs. Batterton approached me first immediately following the worship service, and I knew I was not going to hold up. She's a very special person and she is currently going through chemotherapy. I have tried to be available for them when they needed someone to talk to, but they have not used me much. Well, as others approached, I could not hold back the tears, and then Gwen started crying. I do not want people thinking that I feel bad, or that I am worrying about myself. I'm really not. It is just that I'm very sensitive when others approach me to console me.

As it turned out, radiation was not a cure. The note that follows was the result of me waking up with thoughts running through my head. I was taking chemotherapy treatments for the second time when I wrote the following.

I woke up the morning of June 17, 1998 at 3:30am with the following thoughts. I was wide awake, so I went down stairs and wrote down what I was thinking. Maybe this will let you know more about what's going on in me.

Cancer is a funny thing. It makes me a better person. But "How?" you say?

- It breaks down that huge wall of human pride that keeps me from saying the things people around me need and want to hear.
- It helps me better prioritize what is really valuable in life.
- It is a wake-up call from worldly pride.
- It gives me courage to speak out for things I truly believe in (to voice my true convictions) regardless of the consequence.
- A sense of urgency reappears in my life. Although I've always believed it, it makes it much more clear that there are no guarantees in life.
- I realize that if you have something to say to someone (a loved one in particular), but foolish pride keeps you from 'exposing' your true thoughts, it is time to 'embarrass yourself' and let those you care for hear what you really think.
- I've learned that crying in public is nothing to be ashamed of, but at times I still am.

You pay a price for speaking out, but the cost of holding it in is far greater—endless regret if left unsaid or if unheard by the one who needed it most.

Sometimes the ones that condemn you the most are those who profess to be fellow Christians. Over the last few years that has been a hard lesson for me. If you speak out with God first in mind, when your beliefs are different than your fellow Christians, those fellow Christians can be some of the biggest disappointments in your life because they are the first ones to condemn you. But, God must come first no matter what.

Now, I need to exercise these lessons I say that I have learned. Verbalizing those innermost thoughts comes hard for me. But, if it consoles a loved one when someone on their deathbed expresses their deepest thoughts, how much more it must please their soul to hear or read those words from a healthy person of sound mind. I'll start by putting my thoughts in writing. I'm not emotionally strong enough to speak those 'mushy' words, but at least I can write them down. I have no doubts that I will win this battle, but why run the risk of something else preventing my thoughts from being expressed and those to whom it is intended from hearing them.

After those thoughts, I felt very compelled to express my thoughts to my family. The following is the text that I wrote to each of my loved ones. I share these just to show what helped me deal with cancer, and what was important to me at the time. I'm not trying to show how good I am. Believe me, there were lots of trying times when I was not pleasant to be around.

— — — — — — — — — — — — — — — — — — — —

Dear Gwen,

To the mother of my most cherished blessings, my children. I am very lucky to have such a pretty and understanding wife. You are a beautiful person. I love you very much. I could not be any luckier than to have you for a wife and mother of our children. Although I think at times you are too giving to others, at least I'd rather have you that way, than so self-centered that all you thought about was yourself (that is definitely not a problem).

I know we will make it through these trying times and move on. I appreciate you being there for me, but do not think you always have to be strong for me. If you do not feel strong, do not put on a front. I am strong enough to deal with those things.

I love you,

———————————————————————

Todd,

I am very proud of you. I'm very pleased to see you so confident in yourself and you do have tremendous athletic ability. But, your traits that I like most are:

- Your love for others in that you are not too good to talk to anyone, whether they are black, hispanic, crippled, or retarded.
- You do not 'suck up' to adults or rich friends because you want to be recognized for who you are and what you can do, and
- Your choice of friends most of the time.

You are a good kid. You have brought me years of joy. I'm very strict because I want to keep it that way. Try to understand that. Make sure that God is first in your life. If HE is, other things will fall in place.

Do not worry about me and my bout with cancer. I can handle it with the help of God. I will beat it. But, never think that it cannot happen to you. Always have your heart in the right relationship with God so you do not have to worry.

I love you,

———————————————————————

Garrett,

I see so much of me in you. You are very shy, yet you are a very strong, silent leader. You do not have a lot to say, but I know there's a lot going on in that mind. You 'bottle up' your feelings inside like I do. Learn to express yourself. I do not want it to be hard for you to express yourself like it is for me.

You have brought so much joy to my life. You are a great athlete. It makes me very proud to go to your games and everyone knows you're my son. You showed tremendous courage this year in the way you handled cheerleading and Coach _____. A lot of guys were not as mentally tough as you were. Also, I'm very pleased with the quality of friends you choose.

Do not worry about me and my bout with cancer. I can handle it with the help of God. I will beat it. But, never think that it cannot happen to you. Always have your heart in the right relationship with God so you do not have to worry.

I love you very much,

— — — — — — — — — — — — — — — — — — —

Whitney,

Daddy's little girl ain't so little anymore, but she's precious. Stay innocent and sweet like you are today. I could not have picked anyone as good as I got in you. Everyone loves Whitney and that makes me very proud.

You bring me tremendous joy. I love the relationship that we have developed and I hope it grows.

Do not worry about me and my bout with cancer. I can handle it with the help of God. I will beat it. But, never think that it cannot happen to you. Always have your heart in the right relationship with God so you do not have to worry.

I love you,

———————————————————————————————

When I was diagnosed a second time, I wrote the following memo to my co-workers. Many of them had worked with me when I was diagnosed the first time, but the company had grown and some did not know that I had dealt with cancer in the past.

Memo To Fellow Workers

I am taking the easy way out to update everyone on my health report. I tried to limit the memo mainly to co-workers who where employed when I went through Round 1 in 1993. Feel free to update others that ask that I did not include in the list. I did not exclude anyone for a reason other than new employees wouldn't know the history of my situation.

I went to the doctor this morning to hear the results of my CT scans and to see when treatment would begin, and for how long. Well, the bad news is that I'm not going to die anytime soon from cancer, so there's no immediate relief for you all. You'll have to hire a hit man if you want immediate results. The cancer is currently limited to my neck area. It is a small cell cancer, that they say may pop up from time to time, but it is not the deadly kind if found and treated.

I will have my first chemo on Wednesday afternoon at 2pm. I will have a minimum of 4 treatments and possibly up to 10 treatments. I will have a treatment every 3 weeks. I will be taking 3 of the 4 chemicals I took the first time, but I'm not taking the one drug that causes definite hair loss. I may get to keep some of it. I will be on Prednizone, which is toxic to lymphoma. It will cause me to gain weight and will reshape my head and face for a while. It is the medication my family knows sets me off from time to time—I'm just a little on edge, but the long term effects are for the best. Thanks for all the thoughts and prayers on my behalf.

———————————————————————————

After the third occurrence, we spent five months waiting to decide what was the right course of treatment. There was no rush, since I was dealing with a low-grade lymphoma. It was slow growing, and my options needed to be carefully weighed since my body had already been subjected to two rounds of chemotherapy. Chemotherapy is hard on your body. In particular, the density of my white blood cells had been lessened with each treatment. Because white blood cells are critical for the immune system, we had to carefully decide on the next form of treatment. Finally, I had a CT Scan on May 25th. I had a meeting to discuss the results with my doctor on June 2nd. On June 3rd I was in a great mood. We finally had a plan in place. The waiting to determine the right course of action had been unsettling. I wrote the following email to my brother and his response follows.

Date: Thursday, June 03, 1999 5:50 AM
Subject: CT Scan Update

I did get my test results back yesterday and I did like what I heard. I have 2 nodes that have grown on the right side of my neck. This is the third time in a row that it is only on the right side of the neck, so we are going to cut off my neck. No, we are going to do radiation. Never had that before, but that is what I wanted after we found this in December. Doctor is optimistic that it could be a cure. I do not know that it will work that well for me, but it is a good shot. He is referring me to a doctor in San Marcos today. So it will not be far from work. He thought that radiation would be something like Monday—Friday for 5—6 weeks. It takes about 5-10 minutes to zap you. I'll know more when I meet with the radiation doctor.

My brother's response was:

Great humor! You should keep those first three sentences.

As I mentioned to start this chapter writing was an outlet to me. Express yourself in a way that is easy for you. Others want to know how you are doing, whether good or bad. It is best to not have them guessing all the time. They will feel much better to know how you are doing, and, you will not have the stress of trying to deal with it alone.

Chapter 8

My Background

I was born in Tulsa, Oklahoma. When I was four years old, my parents purchased five acres with a one-bedroom house on it, just outside of Tulsa County. For the next twelve years, my parent's bed was located in the dining room, while my brother and I slept in the bedroom. My brother was eight years older than me, so I had the bedroom to myself from eleven years old on. My mother was a stay-at-home mom until I was thirteen. I think thirteen was the same year that I received my first barbershop haircut. Before that, my mother always gave me a burr haircut. My father worked two jobs—welder by day and a horse trainer in the evenings. My parents finally had enough money to add two bedrooms onto the house, when I was sixteen. It was a very modest life, but we were certainly far from poor as I saw it. Many had it much worse. My parents were just very frugal. Their theory on buying things was if you could not pay cash, you did not need it.

I attended Barnsdall 55, a three-room schoolhouse my first eight years of school. The average enrollment for all eight grades was eighty students. Attending the Barnsdall 55 School in Black Dog Township, in Osage county, was a great time in my life. Everything was so simple. You knew everyone extremely well. In the first grade, I remember having a crush on one of the eighth grade girls. Of course, she never knew it. I was so shy I was not about to tell anyone. My eighth grade graduating class consisted of thirteen students. That was a large class for Barnsdall 55.

I have always loved playing basketball. Although I was probably a better baseball player, basketball was, and is, my first love. We did not have a gymnasium at Barnsdall 55 until I was in the fourth grade. We only had an outside, concrete court. You made the team by making a free throw and that was according to the "honor system." In the second grade, I spent day after day, by myself, for several weeks after school, shooting free throws, until one day I made one. I could not wait for school the next morning, so that I could tell the principal, "I made a free throw." That qualified me for the sixth grade basketball team as a second grader. The school colors at the time were just like the Boston Celtics, Kelly green with white trim. The school colors had been red and white several years before. All of the green uniforms had been handed out, and I was given one of the old red uniforms. That did not matter to me. I was on the team. That was the important part. In the games to follow, I gladly wore that red uniform while my teammates wore their new ones. And, I did play sparingly in the games.

When I graduated from Barnsdall 55, I had the choice of attending one of two large high schools in north Tulsa or attend Sperry High School, which was in Sperry, OK, about six miles north of Tulsa. Sperry was a small community, population about 2,500. My senior class was the largest graduating class to date for Sperry High, with seventy-two graduates in the Class of 1972. High school was a very rewarding time for me. I was a starter in basketball my sophomore, junior and senior years, leading the team in scoring my junior and senior years. I also started in baseball for three years. I was president of my class both as a junior and a senior. During my senior year, I was also the Student Council president. Being enrolled in a small, 2A school provided many opportunities in which to be involved. I still keep in touch with several high school classmates. There is a strong relationship that will always be there. Members of my high school class were shocked to learn of my diagnosis of cancer. I made a couple of trips to Tulsa from Texas to visit them, because they were so encouraging to me. I received numerous phone calls and letters of encouragement from them. Those strong bonds with friends are the most important relationships to have on this earth, outside of our relationship with God and our family.

Gwen and I met on the school bus when I was a freshman. She also had two sisters and a brother that rode the bus. We were good friends for three and one-half years, before we started going steady when I was a senior. During my senior year, on my drive to school each day, I stopped to pick up Gwen and her younger brother so they did not have to endure the long bus ride. During my freshman year in college, we were engaged. Gwen was afraid to break the news to my parents. My father was very angry with me when I told him that I had bought Gwen a ring and that we planned to get married. His life-long dream was that my brother and I would both get a solid college education. My brother had already graduated from college, earned his Master's and passed his CPA exam. My father was afraid that I would not finish my degree, but I knew that I would. During the summers, I had worked too many outside jobs, hauling hay, painting pipe fences, and refinery work, all in the heat, and I knew that I did not want to do manual labor for the rest of my life. I wanted a college degree so that I could have an office job. Gwen and I were married on January 4, 1974, between semesters of my sophomore year in college. I earned my college degree at Oklahoma Sate University in Business Management, while my wife worked. I actually finished my degree in three and one-half years, and my father was pleased. We had little money during those first years of marriage, but we were very happy.

My first job out of college was back in Tulsa at Cities Service Oil Company as a COBOL programmer. Cities Service provided ten weeks of training, teaching me the programming language that provided a living for me. That was tremendous training that I used for the next twenty years and more. They hired people with a college degree. It did not matter what kind of degree you had. The fact that you had persevered and completed your college education with a good GPA was the important factor. Cities Services was committed to providing the work-related training needed to perform your job.

In 1976, Gwen and I bought our first house. It was a small, one thousand square foot house that cost $25,000. Fifteen months later we sold it for $31,000 and bought a larger house in Broken Arrow, OK. Our first son was born in Broken Arrow in 1980. We struggled trying to have a baby, but when he finally arrived, we were elated. Everything was progressing so nicely for us. I had been promoted to branch vice president where I worked. Then in 1983, we hit a minor bump in the road when that company filed for bankruptcy, but that provided me with an opportunity to enter into a partnership with a fellow employee. I always had a strong desire to have my own business. This situation pushed me to start my own business. Our small company struggled and I stayed with it for seven years, but it was always a challenge to maintain a steady income stream. And, I'm not talking about a nice income. My salary went from $38,000 in 1983 to $23,000 in 1984, but I was doing what I wanted to do in trying to build a business. Things were still progressing much to my satisfaction. I had always dreamed of building my own business and providing financial security for my family. Financial security was just a dream. To supplement our income, I was a basketball referee for several years. Those seven years of self-employment satisfied that thirst to be my own boss. If I had never tried it, I would probably still have that lingering need to try it, but my health conditions would keep me from pursuing it.

Chapter 9

I Asked for a Change—Boy Did I Get It!

In the early 90's, my life was frustrating to me. I was bored. I needed "change" in my life! My career was not going the way I had planned for it to go. At work, I felt that I deserved to be in a management position, but I had philosophical differences with the department head. I could not foresee achieving my goals by remaining with my current employer, so I started looking for a management opportunity with other companies. I guess I was a little too general in my wish for change. I'll warn you now, do not ask for something, unless you know you want it, because you may just get what you ask for, and more. It seemed like our married life had progressed in a pretty typical, middle-class, American style. We were not able to have children as soon as we would have liked to, but we ended up with three healthy children by the time I was thirty years of age. I was never without a job, although I did become self-employed as a result of the employer going bankrupt. In 1989, I went back to work for a large corporation. Self-employment for me was a very stressful time, without much reward. My business partner did not have the same work ethic that I had, nor was he punctual. Foolishly, I thought that I could change him, but that was so wrong. After doing everything I could to make it work, I finally came to the realization that it was not worth the numerous hours that it kept me from my family.

In 1992, without mentioning it to Gwen, I really started thinking about moving away from Tulsa, Oklahoma. Although we had lived the last seventeen years in Broken Arrow, that was just a bedroom community to Tulsa. I had worked at the same place since July 1989. Opportunities for advancement into management had come and gone without any changes for me. I wanted a 'change' in my life. I was born in Tulsa, Oklahoma, in 1954, and except for about a year and a half of living in Stillwater, OK, while working to attain my college degree, I had spent my entire life in or near Tulsa.

Maybe it was a 'mid-life crisis' that I was starting to go through. For whatever reason, I was tired of Tulsa. I did not like the climate; the size of the local school district; the pace at which my career was advancing, nor living close to my parents. My excuse was that I did not want my children thinking that they had to spend their lives living close to Mom and Dad out of duty, especially if they did not want to do so. I wanted to set an example for my children, so I kept searching for a way to satisfy my needs and be an example at the same time. In June 1992, I learned that there was a company in Texas that was contemplating the possibility of buying the software that I had worked on during the last three years. After talking to a couple of fellow workers, I submitted a resume to the company in Texas. Three weeks later, Gwen and I were flying to New Braunfels, Texas for an interview and a weekend to look over the area. Gwen had no intentions of moving from Tulsa. All of her family lived there and she did not want to move away, but she was willing to let me search it out. I do not believe she ever thought that we would really move. I had never been any further south in Texas than Dallas. My expectations did not match up with what we saw and experienced on the trip. I expected to find the following in San Antonio—a flat, dry, land with cactus and tumbleweeds rolling around. When we arrived at the airport it was late on a Friday evening, so I could not see the layout of the area into which we had just flown. We got up early Saturday morning and drove from San Antonio up to New Braunfels. Much to our surprise, we could not find anything negative about the area. It was green, with rolling hills and plenty of trees. It was not at all what we had expected to find. It was much nicer than anything we had pictured. After a short interview that morning, we spent the rest of the weekend looking around New Braunfels. On Saturday evening, some people took us to a Mexican restaurant in downtown San Antonio, then on to the River Walk. We had a great time. We really liked what we saw, and it looked like the company was interested in hiring me.

Three weeks later, I flew to the company headquarters in Abilene, Texas, for a second interview with the president of the company. The flight there was uneventful, which is always a good thing when you are flying. We had a good day and we were able to come to an agreement that I would be hired into a management position. The flight back to Dallas was a different story. I had to fly from Abilene to Dallas in a small, 15-seat plane. There were thunderstorms all around Dallas. The flight was short, but not nearly short enough. The pilot tried to fly around the storm, but we entered into a lot of turbulence. As you can tell by now though, I made it home.

The decision was final! We were moving our family to New Braunfels, Texas. Based on that decision, I was not a very popular person with my family. Gwen was my only support. Gwen sure did not want to leave her family nor our church family, but being the good, understanding wife that she was, she was willing to let me do what I felt was best. My kids did not want to leave all of their friends, schools and sports teams. There was a great deal of comfort in their everyday life. They knew who their friends where. They knew what teachers they liked and which ones they did not like. For the most part, they knew who their teammates would be on the next basketball, softball or baseball team, also knowing that they would be playing the positions that they wanted to play. Church was a place where my children had many friends very similar in age. They had grown up with those friends and families. We had attended the same church for their entire lifetimes, up to that point. My children did not like the idea of moving, but my parents hated it! They could not believe that I (their baby) would uproot my family and move five hundred miles away. As far as they were concerned, I had all I needed in my current job. It was a good paying job. I was receiving promotions and pay increases from time-to-time in Tulsa, and leaving that job was foolishness in their minds. Their question was "Why in the world would you leave something like that?" I could not be completely honest with my parents in answering that question. One of the main reasons that I wanted to leave was to put a significant distance between my immediate family and my parents. My parents were smothering me! We could never give them enough time to satisfy them. They exerted constant pressure on us to drive out to their house every weekend. It was their expectation. This topic is discussed in greater detail a little later.

My parents did not want to understand certain circumstances, nor were they willing to try to understand my desires and goals in life. I was the younger of two children. My brother was still living in Tulsa at the time, so I was the first in the family to move away. Three of the five grandchildren were my children, and the announcement that I was moving them far away was not acceptable. So why did I move the family? It was probably because I was selfish. This was something 'I' really wanted to do. In fact, there were specific things that I wanted to do. For years, I had an urge to move, but I never felt that I could do so and keep the family happy. I felt constrained by my parents that somehow they would not understand why I felt such a need to leave 'home'. My feeling was accurate. Secondly, I wanted to demonstrate to my children that they would not have to feel the same pressures that I had felt from my parents. They should be ready to move and not feel guilty if they have a tremendous opportunity that would require them to move far away from us (Mom and Dad). Finally, I wanted to move out of Broken Arrow, because it was the largest school district in Oklahoma. I believed that being able to play school sports would be one of the most rewarding things in my children's lives. I did not want to take the chance of them doing that in Broken Arrow. They were young, and that was of no concern to them, but I wanted to provide them with the best opportunity in the years ahead. I attended small schools—one with a total of eighty children enrolled, and then my high school only had seventy-two in my class. I knew that I was able to participate at a high level in a small school, and I had real concerns about their opportunities in a large school, because there can be so many good athletes turned away in a large school.

One of the major risks I had taken was that we had to sell our house ourselves. My new employer was not going to purchase our home, and the real estate market in Broken Arrow, OK, was at best, weak. We immediately contracted with a real estate agent and placed our house on the market. The asking price for our house was about $5,500 more than we had paid for the house seven years earlier. During that time we had made numerous improvements to the house, including installing siding, which cost $7,500. Needless to say, we knew that we were going to lose some money on the sale. That was acceptable though, because I really wanted to make a move, to 'shake up' my life. I just did not have a clue how much it would be shaken. My job started in Texas on August 24, 1992, so I commuted between New Braunfels and Tulsa for about two and one-half months. Gwen and I had a very strong marriage, so we knew that we could handle the distance. Finally, in October, someone was interested in the house and made us an offer. The offer was much lower than our asking price, but there were not any other offers to consider. It was a reasonable offer, so we took it. Two and one-half months of commuting and only seeing your family for a weekend every two weeks is very trying on a strong relationship, much less a weak one. I would never recommend it to any other couple. Of course, we were not the first to do it, nor will we be the last. The only difference is that I chose to do it because 'I wanted to', not because I was forced to do it.

First of all, let me tell you about "the move." In the week prior to moving to Texas, we had just returned from the Mickey Mantle / Whitey Ford Fantasy camp. The only negative result from the camp was the fact that I broke my left wrist. My left arm was in a cast. That was a challenge since I was the person loading the remaining items into a rental truck. A moving company was responsible for moving the main items in our house, but we still rented a small truck for plants and collectible items that we did not want to leave in the hands of others. I was able to load the truck, even with the cast on my left arm. We started the trip to Texas on Saturday morning, November 21, about 10:30 a.m. We wanted to get away sooner, but neighbors and friends kept stopping by to say their good-byes. At the same time, a winter storm with snow was heading south into Oklahoma, so we needed to get on the road. We left wearing our shorts, knowing that we were headed south to Texas where it was very warm. I drove the rental truck and our dog, Shadow, rode with me. Gwen and the kids rode in the van. They were crying when we left, because their lives were starting to change, but at the same time, they were laughing at me, because the dog and I had to ride together. Shadow and I were not the best of friends, so that was funny to everyone except me. At the same time, I knew that I could not say much since I was forcing them to move.

We were on the road about three hours, when Gwen pulled up along side of the truck as we were driving down the interstate, and she signaled for me to pull over at the next place for a rest stop. Remember, this was back in 1992 and we did not have a cell phone then. How things have changed! Anyway, I took the next exit, and when I did, I noticed that I could not accelerate. As the truck had tried to downshift gears (it was an automatic transmission), apparently the gearing broke. The truck coasted into the parking lot of the convenience store, and I called for service. The service people agreed to find another truck, bring it to our location, and we would switch trucks. Now remember, we were about two hours ahead of a winter storm when we left home. We sat down at a table in the convenience store, and the kids mentioned that they were hungry. We purchased two sandwiches and cold drinks. Our middle son could not finish his sandwich, so Mom (Gwen) decided to finish it. After eating it and killing time, out of sheer boredom she started reading the sandwich wrapper. She noticed that the expiration date had passed by about two weeks, but it was too late. The sandwich tasted fine, so she really did not think anymore about it. So, after eating, we continued to sit around, waiting on the other truck. Here came the winter storm. The wind started blowing hard, and the temperature plummeted. Finally, after a three hour wait, they drove up in another rental truck. By that time, the winter storm had caught up with us. It was snowing; the wind was cutting through us, and we had to transfer all of the stuff from the broken down truck into the replacement truck. Luckily, when I opened the back of the truck, we found that one of the bags that we had thrown into the truck at the last minute was full of ski jackets and hats. That was pure luck. At least we had some warm coats to wear. The men that brought the truck and I began to transfer the load from one truck to the other. My broken arm was tested again, but that was not a big deal. By now, it was 4:30 in the afternoon, and we still had at least 6 hours of travel time left. At least we were back on the road. Two and a half hours down the road, Gwen pulled the van up along side the truck and told me that we needed to find an exit immediately. We pulled over at the next exit, and she explained to me that Garrett was sick. His stomach was aching and he was vomiting. Guess what? Food poisoning. We pulled back onto the interstate and forty-five minutes later, she needed to pull over again. Gwen looked into our ice chest. Fortunately, when she was emptying the refrigerator, she had put some medication in the ice chest. She gave some to Garrett. We got back on the interstate and continued south. A little over an hour later, Gwen pulled beside me and said we need to pull over again. Now, both Gwen and Garrett were really hurting. She would have felt a lot better if we could have just found a hotel for the night, but I needed to get to New Braunfels. I was scheduled to leave on a business trip at 1 p.m. on Sunday afternoon. I had a presentation to make at a customer's site in St. Louis on Monday morning. There was a major sales opportunity for my employer. I was the person that knew the most about the new software and there was no option, but for me to go! Finally, we pulled into our hotel in New Braunfels at about 1:30 a.m. We got to sleep in our room about 2:30 a.m., and Gwen and Garrett felt horrible. The only good news was that it was easy to sneak the dog into the room at that hour of the night. Early the next morning, I called the airlines and scheduled a later flight out on Sunday afternoon. Both Garrett and Gwen felt weak, but better after a night's sleep. Gwen took me to the airport on Sunday afternoon. I had to leave my family in a new town, feeling sick and not knowing anyone. I was able to return late on Monday night. This occurred the week of Thanksgiving, so our kids did not miss much school that week.

The following week, the kids started school in Texas. Gwen had always been involved with the PTA at our children's elementary school. Now, she did not have a clue about what went on in the new school. It took about three months to get to know any friends. In January, our boys started playing in the city basketball program. That provided an opportunity for them to meet new friends, but more importantly, it allowed Gwen and me to meet other parents. The baseball season provided more opportunities to meet new friends. Just when we started feeling comfortable in our new environment, I was diagnosed with cancer. Of course, my job stability was a huge concern. I had only been with the company for six months, and now I had cancer. My fear was, "How is my employer going to handle this situation?" It was the first time that the small company had faced a major health issue with an employee. Fortunately, my job was not in jeopardy. I wanted a change in my life—I got one! It was not what I had pictured, though.

Once you are diagnosed with cancer, your life will never be the same again. Mine certainly has not been the same, and by most accounts, the changes have been for the better. I look at life with a totally different view, which includes more appreciation for the little things, and a stronger commitment to follow the Word of God.

Very seldom does a day go by without me thinking about having, or having had cancer. It is not that I pity myself, nor do I fear dying from cancer. It is simply a reminder that life is such a precious commodity. I rarely take a day in my life for granted. When my sons or daughter visit home, then when they get ready to leave, I know that I may never see them again, so I always tell them how much I love them. I do not assume that I will be here tomorrow, and I recognize that their lives are not guaranteed either. I want to make sure that if I die, my children know that their father loved them. If they were to be in a car accident, I do not want to put myself in the situation of regretting that I did not assure them that I loved them.

When we are always healthy, it is very easy to take life for granted. You expect that you can do this or that tomorrow.

Our health is not a consideration, because we assume that we will be just as fit tomorrow as we are today. So, I do not view living with an illness as a dreaded burden. There are many positive benefits.

What was so positive? I am more focused on my spiritual life, realizing that my life could be taken at any time, so I better have things in order at all times. Now, that does not mean that I do not slip at times. I have weak moments like anyone else, but I have many more strong times than weak times. I appreciate each and every day of my life. I understand that it is not a given that I will have tomorrow, so I need to make the most of each day. I verbalize my true love for my family much more than before. When friends or acquaintances are diagnosed with cancer, I have a much better understanding of the issues and decisions they face, and I want to provide comfort to them. Gwen is much more comforting than I am, because she has been through the struggles of cancer as a spouse. She has a different perspective than I do. My children have grown much stronger emotionally, because of this challenge. All of these things are positive results from my cancer.

Following the diagnosis and treatments, I have become a very emotional person. There are times when I cannot control my tears. Why, I am not sure. Others expressing their concern for my family, or complementing my children has become so meaningful. At first, it was not easy for me to openly cry in front of others at work or church. But, I did not have any control of my emotions. In many ways, I am still that way. If I am listening to someone explain hard times that they have experienced, I become very empathetic with them. It is very difficult for me to keep from crying. It is also very hard for me to verbalize my compassion for them and express concern to that individual sharing the story, because I cannot talk without being emotional. This impacts another part of my life as well. For entertainment, Gwen and I like to go to movies.

Controlling my tears in sad scenes, emotional scenes, or even those scenes where someone is expressing their love for their children is not an option that I can control. Gwen and I just cry together during the movies. Gwen no longer gets embarrassed over her tears, because I am doing the same thing.

Chapter 10

Mental Toughness

Our strong faith in God is what gets us through the difficult times. I was thirty-nine years old when I was first diagnosed with cancer. Through my school years, college and work, I had always been extremely active in sports, playing softball and basketball, plus coaching my children's basketball, baseball and softball. It was nothing for me to be playing softball four nights a week, on two different leagues. Then on the weekends, there were tournaments. Between those games I was coaching baseball or softball. There was not much time spent in front of television, because my schedule was so full of activities. I have never abused my body in any way, not with alcohol, drugs or tobacco. The worst things that I had put in my body were Twinkies and Peeps Easter candy. My close friends were in shock when they learned that I had cancer. They recognized how "clean" and healthy a life I had lived, and they were just amazed that I had cancer.

Six months prior to my first cancer diagnosis, I had uprooted my family and moved them to Texas, five hundred miles from any family. Other than for the few people that I knew at my new job, we were alone. We did not know anyone in our new community. We were starting anew—different house, new town and state, new job, new schools, new church. My family was dealing with new surroundings, trying to make new friends and then we found out I had cancer. What a shock! It was an extremely stressful time for us. Obviously, this news was not the only thing impacting our lives. Everything was in flux!

At the time that my cancer was diagnosed my parents lived five hundred miles away and they had no clue that I was going to have surgery. Gwen and I were not going to alarm them over the removal of a simple cyst. It was no big deal, right? So we thought. Immediately after the surgery, everything changed. The doctor informed Gwen of his shocking discovery. She later informed me. When I learned of it, all kinds of questions filled my head. Was the surgeon certain that he had found cancer during the surgery? If so, how do you break the news to your parents over the phone that you have cancer? It is not an easy thing to do, but anyone faced with this situation, has to do the same thing. How long do you wait to tell them? Do you keep it to yourself for a while? Do you call them immediately after leaving the doctor's office? More importantly, how do you break the news to your children? What kind of impact would this have on my children? When do we tell them? How long will I be alive? How is this going to impact my job? Am I going to be able to work during the treatments? Cancer was a very frightening situation for us, because my niece had a near death experience a few years earlier.

Question after question pops into your head after this kind of news. Initially, you are overwhelmed. But after gathering our thoughts, Gwen and I remembered God and the promises that he has made to those who are faithful to him. That is a very comforting feeling. It takes some time to get past being overwhelmed with concern and turning to God. However, it is your most important destination on your roller coaster ride of emotions. Focusing on your spiritual life can be both peaceful and haunting, though. If you have not been faithful to God; if your life has been focused on everything except your obedience to God, then it can be very haunting. You can become overwhelmed with despair. Thankfully, if you are a Christian, you have the hope of prayer. If you have been striving to follow God's Word, then it will be peaceful. I have been in both situations and those are the ways in which I was impacted. Speaking with God through prayer will always help you to deal with these trying situations. When you do not want others to know, or you do not want to immediately ask for their help, God is always there for you. God is the One on whom you can depend. Friends may be consumed in their own lives. God always has time for you, and is waiting for you to ask for help. In **II Corinthians 1:3, 4 (KJV)**, Paul tells how God provided comfort as he labored in the Word. We have that same promise of comfort as Christians.

II Cor. 1:3 Blessed *be* the God and Father of our Lord Jesus Christ, the Father of mercies and God of all comfort, **4** who comforts us in all our tribulation, that we may be able to comfort those who are in any trouble, with the comfort with which we ourselves are comforted by God.

In **Matthew 11:28—30 (KJV)**, Jesus was teaching disciples. He taught the following.

His words are very comforting. His offer is available to everyone.

Matt. 11:28 Come to Me, all *you* who labor and are heavy laden, and I will give you rest. **29** Take My yoke upon you and learn from Me, for I am gentle and lowly in heart, and you will find rest for your souls. **30** For My yoke *is* easy and My burden is light.

Dealing with cancer has made us stronger people—stronger in facing adversity; stronger in dealing with tragedy and difficult situations. For one thing, it taught us how to depend on God to help us get through difficult times. Second, when facing a difficult situation, I always remind myself that things could still be much worse than they are at the present time. Gwen and I are still here to support one another. Our children are still very healthy. Just in those two statements, it is easy to see how much worse things could be. I could lose Gwen to a car accident, or she could be stricken with cancer herself. One or more of our children could be killed in a drive-by shooting, or hit by a drunk driver as they are riding in a car. Another member of our family could be dealing with a terminal illness, but none are. The list could go on and on about all the potential diseases or accidents that could occur. There is no doubt that things could be much worse.

You will find Gwen or me making jokes when we are confronted with a new tragedy. Comments like, "Well, you are not going to believe this, but something bad has happened again." Or, we might say, "Guess what happened this time?" That kind of humor has also helped us to remain strong in times of problems. It has gotten to the point where Gwen becomes uncomfortable when our lives appear simple and smooth. The question becomes, "What is lurking around the corner for us?" It is almost like we have become accustomed to dealing with stressful situations and for things to not be that way is strange. Gwen sent me an email one day that was offering us family training on how to cope with the daily stress in our lives. I replied to her email with, "We don't need to go. We could be teaching that class." In that response, I was not meaning that the training would not be valuable for people. I just believed that we did not need to spend $100 on that particular training, based on our many experiences. That is just an example of the humor that we use to defuse stress.

Chapter 11

The Flood

The river started coming over its banks about 12:45 p.m. on Saturday afternoon, October 17, 1998. It had rained steadily all morning, but the thought of a flood never entered our mind. About 11:00 a.m., Garrett called and said that he needed to be picked up at the high school. The team had been viewing football films from the previous night's game. Eleven a.m. was much earlier than usual for the session to end, but he said that the school parking lot was starting to flood and they were stopping early so the players could get home safely. When I picked Garrett up, we drove to get haircuts. We encountered intersections containing deep waters. Our course had to be changed a couple of times. But, we got our haircuts and returned home safely, so we just thought that there had been a lot of rain—no big deal. By 1:30 p.m., flood waters starting creeping into our front yard. I was still so naïve. I did not think there was any way that our house was going to flood. The boys and I had spent the past forty-five minutes moving all of my baseball memorabilia from under the stairway downstairs, up to the master bedroom. I just knew with certainty that it would all be safe upstairs. How wrong I was!

Gwen and Whitney had spent that forty-five minutes knocking on neighbors' doors and warning them of the rising waters. At one house, they were unaware of what was going on prior to Gwen knocking on their door. Their parents were gone and the children were not paying any attention to the weather, because they were watching Saturday morning cartoons. They were very thankful for the warning. Shortly after 1:30 p.m. we loaded up two of our cars and started up the hill—the only way out of the neighborhood. On the way out of the house, Gwen grabbed our video camera that was sitting on the kitchen table. It had a charged battery in it, because she had taken it to the football game the night before, however, she did not do much filming. In disbelief, we started to drive out of the neighborhood. Gwen had me stop while she recorded the rising waters for a few minutes. Before she got back into the car, the first policeman arrived to warn us. Gwen responded to the policeman, "Where have you been?" His response was that they had been going through the neighborhoods warning people for several hours, and he was the first to reach our area. The police had been working hard, but we were not aware of it until then. We proceeded to drive over to one of our friend's house to spend the afternoon. We planned to return home that evening with no problem, or possibly a muddy garage. We ended up spending the next fifteen days living with Rita and her family. When we left our house, we thought that the water might get into our garage, and that would be that. We left with just the clothes on our back, and two of our three vehicles, the video camera and our two outside dogs. Time was a huge factor and we only had two drivers at home. We took the two vehicles that had the highest ground clearance. Our new car, that was less than a month old, was left in our garage. That is how confident we were that nothing major would happen. And, that shows how foolish and ignorant we were.

During that afternoon, Gwen frequently called one of our neighbors who remained in the neighborhood. Their house was one of only three spared from any water damage. When Gwen first called about 2:30 p.m., our neighbor said that the water was in our first floor. That was shocking and it sounded bad, but we could live with that. About an hour later, she called and our neighbor said that the water was in our second story. Gwen responded, "No way!" He assured her that he saw just that. When she got off the phone, she called our family into a bedroom and told everyone the news she had just learned. Garrett was the first to go to pieces crying. All he could think about was our bird. He had taken the birdcage up to the master bedroom and placed it on the floor, where he thought it would be safe. Then, all he could think about was the bird drowning. That sounds so simple, but that was devastating to him.

By 5:00 p.m., floodwaters had risen to seventeen feet in our house, about thirty inches above the second-story floor. The rains ended about that time. We drove back over to our neighborhood. We lived in a low-lying area, down a steep hill, with a twenty-one percent grade. We parked at the top of the hill, and walked about two-thirds of the way down. Several of our neighbors were there also. We shared tears and stories with each other. All you could see were the rooftops poking out of the water. To the far left, the river was roaring, and we heard the crackling sound of massive trees being snapped as complete houses rushed by. That was a very sobering site. Seeing the home that you were just in five hours earlier, now barely peaking above the cresting waters that engulfed it, caused you to have extremely lost, insecure and very emotional feelings. We had to go to the store that evening to purchase clothes, toothbrushes, hair brushes, contact lens solution, shampoo and dog food. As stated earlier, we had left the house with only the clothes on our backs.

We were able to enter the house the following morning about 8:30 a.m. Gwen and I woke up at sunrise, before anyone else, and drove over to our house. The waters had receded and the streets, yards, and driveways were covered with four to eight inches of mud. We could not believe our eyes. When we left on Saturday afternoon, the yards were alive, full of vibrant colors, especially the huge, pink crepe myrtle trees in our front yard. Sunday morning, it was brown, solid mud covering the streets, yards, fields and driveways, with a silence like we had never heard. Debris covered the vacant lots and was dangling high up in the trees. As we got out of our car, a policeman drove by and stopped to see who we were. We told him that it was our house and we came to see the damage. He told us that all of the electricity was turned off, but I looked and saw that our landscape lights were still lit. Before leaving the house, I never thought about turning off the main power to the house. So that was my first task before we tried to enter the house. Then, we had some difficulty getting in. The door locks were corroded and full of mud. We could not get a key in the lock. In a matter of hours, corrosion had occurred, plus deposits of mud appeared in every crevice. I had to find a screwdriver to take off the back storm door by removing the hinges. We were finally able to enter our home about an hour later. To go inside and see all of your furniture, electronics and pictures ruined was very disheartening. But, what made me break down and cry was to see all of the pictures of our children as babies strewn all over the stairway, ruined by the waters.

It was difficult to maneuver through our kitchen. The center island had been ripped from the floor and was on it is side. The refrigerator had toppled onto it. The breakfast table and chairs were all over the place. At the same time, it was amazing how some things never moved. My work pager was still on top of the microwave where I had left it. Why didn't it float away? Canisters were full of water, but sat in their usual spots on the counter. We had gone to the grocery store a few days earlier and our pantry was fully stocked. Everything in there was ruined. As the day warmed up, the smell got worse and worse.

We tried to enter the garage, but the door would barely open. When we pried at the door, we could see that the freezer was on top of our new car that we had left in the garage. Remember, prior to leaving, I "knew" that just a little bit of water would reach the garage. Wrong! All of the shelves had come off the walls. The ceiling sheetrock had fallen. Everything in the attic had fallen into the garage, or was hanging. Mud was very deep in there as well. Our garage door was partially raised, which allowed all of our Christmas decorations to be removed with the receding waters.

Next we walked inside the house and up the stairs to the second floor. We started calling for our bird, Rocky, and looking for Todd's pet iguana. The bird was not responding, chirping back, as he normally would. Then we saw his birdcage on its side. The door of the cage was open, and he was out, but where? We looked and looked, but could not find him. Later, Gwen called and told Garrett that we could not find the bird. He responded by telling Mom, "Don't worry about it, Mom." She said, "What?" Then he replied, "Don't tell Dad, but Todd has Rocky." So, Gwen just kept it to herself.

Then there were all of my baseball cards, autographed baseballs, and other memorabilia on the upstairs floor. They were all ruined. A few things were on our bed and some were salvaged, but not much. The bed mattress was completely saturated with water; so many things on top of the bed were ruined. I estimated my sports memorabilia loss was at least $60,000. I had been collecting for years. For the last five years, it was a hobby that I shared with my sons. The loss was sickening, but the fact was that it was all ruined and there was nothing that I could do about it, so it was time to move on. Gwen and I held each other, shedding tears and reminding ourselves that all of it was just "things." The important thing was that we still had our family and friends and we would get through this. We did not have a clue how, without flood insurance to help, but we knew with God's help, we would get by. I went outside while Gwen filmed the inside of the house with the video camera. I didn't have a clue as to where to start.

About six inches of mud covered the driveway, sidewalks and yard. I found a shovel and started shoveling the mud off the driveway. I knew that we needed a place to set all of the stuff as we removed it from the house. Before I was very far along, friends started showing up. It felt great to have our friends come and help. At the same time, I probably was not as receptive as I should have been, mainly because I was in shock. People kept arriving and asking, "What do you want me to do?" I was not of the mindset to put together a plan and delegate responsibilities to others. I knew that everyone wanted to help, but I had a very difficult time telling them what to do. For one thing, I was overwhelmed with the whole situation. I think that Gwen probably did a better job coordinating everyone, and that was a role reversal for us. I typically am a "take charge" person who is well organized. At that particular time, I just wanted to physically work through the pain and disbelief. I continued to shovel mud. I piled it off to the sides of the driveway. That ended up being a pile of mud that was eighteen inches deep and about three feet wide on either side of the driveway. Later, I wished that I had not piled it on my yard. It was a real mess to clean up a couple of months later, because it dried up and crusted over like concrete. We spent the day dragging furniture out of the house and rinsing it off on the driveway, if it was possibly salvageable. Mattresses were laid on the grass, end-to-end, from the front sidewalk to the driveway as a trail for workers.

On Sunday evening, when we returned to our friends' house, the boys revealed to us that they had Rocky. It turned out that Todd and a friend borrowed a canoe; sneaked down the hill at the back of the neighborhood, past the National Guard; placed the canoe in the water and rowed to the back of our house, the night of the flood, about dusk. They said that the water was almost level with Todd's bedroom window sill on the second story. Todd had left his bedroom window unlocked. He rowed up to it, raised the window and climbed into the house. He was determined to rescue the pets. In searching for the bird, he entered Garrett's room where the console television was upended in the water. Upon stepping into the room, Todd was immediately shocked and struggled to get to the bed. He said that it was like stepping on glass. Because the electricity was never turned off, he was receiving electrical currents through the water. Finally, he was able to jump onto the bed. His legs were aching from the shock. Later his fingernails actually turned black on the ends of the fingers, because of the electricity that ran through his body. Eventually, Todd was able to exit the room by climbing on furniture, and get to the master bedroom, where he found Rocky clinging to a towel in the bathroom. He rescued Rocky by placing him in a shoebox; searched for and found his iguana, then exited the house. He was getting ready to leave when he heard the neighbors' cat meowing in a tree, so he stopped and rescued it as well. Later, he told stories about how eerie it was to see so many of our personal items that were normally kept downstairs, floating at the top of the stairway. He recalled hearing the dull sound of an alarm going off, and lights dimly flashing in the deep water as they rowed along. As he got close, he discovered that it was a car submerged in the water. Remember, the waters were seventeen feet deep at that time. Needless to say, I was not aware of his actions for several days. It was kept from me, for fear of how I might respond.

Earlier, I told you about us returning to the top of the hill on Saturday afternoon. By the time we left, it was starting to get dark. As we drove away, Gwen and I saw Todd and his friend walking, carrying a canoe. We specifically told them to stay away from the water, because it was too dangerous. Of course, they responded, "Alright, we won't go down there." But, we know the end of this story. We soon learned they had disobeyed us, because of their concern for the pets. After it was all over and I was told the story a few days later, I did not scold him for going against my orders. There were too many more important issues on my mind. That was one battle I chose to not fight. He was safe and healthy. We had all suffered many losses and that was what he thought that he needed to do. He had witnessed how upset Garrett was when he first thought that the bird was going to die, so Todd was doing it for his brother. It was not the right thing to do, but I understood why he did it. My reaction was the result of lessons that I have learned from dealing with cancer—don't sweat the small stuff, and learn to pick your battles.

The National Guard had men stationed at the entrance to our subdivision to keep "sightseers" and looters out, and to allow the homeowners and their friends to work. Gwen had to leave the house to get some cleaning supplies on Sunday afternoon. When she returned to the neighborhood, she stopped to inform the guard who she was, and he responded, "Oh! You are the folks with all the volunteers coming to help!" When she arrived at the house, she came and told me what the man had said. That was such a comforting feeling. What a humbling message! It made us stop and realize how blessed we were to have such thoughtful, loving friends. Even in this time of tremendous stress and pressures, it was obvious that things could be much worse. We could see neighbors that had no one helping them. There were even people who we did not know that stopped and wanted to help us. We thanked them and told them about the other flood victims who had no help. We sent some of our volunteers toward an area where senior citizens needed help.

Gwen and I really enjoy our friendships. We love doing things with people from church and with the parents of our children's friends. Those friendships were our salvation during those trying times. Several teenagers who were friends of our children came and helped in the cleanup. Friends brought their trucks and trailers to haul off our furniture. Things that could be salvaged were placed in friends' garages and barns. We had things in so many places that we forgot about a lot of things, until we ran into those people months later.

Then there was my cousin Bob. He was a cousin by marriage, not blood-kin (but who cares) that showed up every day at our house to help clean up for three weeks. I only stated "not blood kin" to emphasize the magnitude of his giving; his depth of service to us. To me, it emphasizes the true love that he showed by always being there for us, even though he had only been part of our family for a relatively short time. Bob had to drive about 45 miles each way. When I had to go back to work, Gwen and Bob spent all day working around the house. They used a pressure washer over and over, to remove the mud and bacteria. There was not much that I could do in the evenings, because it got dark too early and there was no electricity to the house. Bob will always have a very special place in our hearts.

Chapter 12

My Brother's Sudden Death

In April 1999, my parents moved from Tulsa, Oklahoma to New Braunfels, Texas. They had decided that their five-acre homestead in Tulsa was too much for my father to maintain at his age. My brother and I had both moved from Tulsa and my parents felt that it was time to move closer to one of us. Since I was the "unhealthy son", my mother asked if it would be okay if they moved to New Braunfels. My mother wanted to be closer to me so she could help take care of me. I thought about my mother's question and answered, "Sure, that is fine." I recognized that they were getting up in years, and it would be much easier for me to care for them if they lived close to me. At the same time, I knew that there would be some real challenges with them living close to us again. To say that I was not excited about them moving was a gross understatement. I dreaded the move. My family had enjoyed our seven years of living five hundred plus miles from my parents. We enjoyed a lot of freedom in that long-distance relationship. One of the main reasons that I moved from Tulsa in the first place was to get away from my parents. I felt smothered with their love and demands while living so close to them. I want to qualify my comments—I had good parents. They were very caring and family was the most important thing in their lives. I just wanted independence a lot more than they wanted me to have it.

My brother, Gary, was eight years older than me. In our younger years, we were not always close because of our age difference. After he turned sixteen, he was gone most of the summers working out of town. When he went off to college, he did not return home very often, and my parents did not travel to Stillwater to see him either. For several years, we simply did not see much of each other. Many years later, after I had graduated from college and began to work in Tulsa things changed for the best. Our relationship started to grow stronger. We were probably closer than we had ever been at the time that I decided to accept the job in Texas. My brother and I enjoyed going to college basketball games in the winter. We both graduated from Oklahoma State University, plus we both lived in the Tulsa area, so we followed Tulsa University and OSU sports. We also attended some college baseball games. At one point, he had season tickets to the Tulsa Ice Oilers, so we attended several hockey games together. My point is, we were very close and did a lot of things together. When I was diagnosed with cancer, he was very active in doing research and providing me with informational resources. If I needed something, I could go to him. He was an awesome "big brother."

On June 27, 1999, we were moving back into our house after it had been rebuilt, following the flood. A family from church was helping us that afternoon. Our friends had their three children with them. It was a joy to have young children, full of excitement and laughter, in our house again. One of our main tasks for the day was to get the clothes washer and dryer operational. That is always important in a family with three teenagers. We had just completed the hook-up of the appliances when I received a phone call from my sister-in-law in Scottsdale, Arizona about 6:00 p.m. She sounded very tired and shaken. She asked if I was sitting down. With that question, I knew that the news could not be good, but I had no idea just how bad the news would be. She proceeded to tell me that she and my brother had been hiking that morning and my brother became very ill. To make a long story short, he was overtaken with heat stroke and died before they could get him to a hospital. My brother and his wife had moved to Scottsdale about two years earlier. They had a beautiful home and were enjoying life. My brother and his wife often went on hikes. Shortly before that, we had visited them in April. My brother paid for our trip. He felt that we needed a little rest and relaxation from the stress of the flooded house and the return of my cancer. Shortly after that, he and his wife came to New Braunfels in May to celebrate my father's eightieth birthday. My brother was fifty-two and appeared to be very healthy. We had a great visit during that trip. My brother was the happiest that I had ever known him to be. He loved living in Scottsdale. He loved working for his employer and was so excited to drive us around the area, to show us their projects in progress. Then one month later, that dreaded phone call came. My sister-in-law asked if I could go over to my parents' house to deliver the bad news and be with them. That was the only right way for it to be done, but wow! I have never dreaded anything so much in my life! How do you tell your parents that their oldest son has died? I sure had no experience in that. At the same time, I know that I am not the first person to ever have that daunting task. I'm just expressing how dreadful a task that it was, and I can certainly empathize with anyone who has to deliver a message like that to his or her parents.

After I put down the phone, I delivered the devastating news to Gwen and our friends. Our friends left shortly after that. Gwen and I drove over to my parents' house late that Sunday evening. That in itself was unusual. They were surprised to see us drive up. My dad greeted us outside, and we went into their house. At that time, I was very well composed. I had not cried at all about my brother's death. Remember, I have written earlier about how emotional I had become ever since my initial diagnosis of cancer. In this particular case, I believe that I was so shocked, that it just did not appear to be real. I asked my parents to come into the living room and sit down. They knew something was wrong. I told them that I had some very bad news. I then explained that my sister-in-law had called and that my brother, their son, had died from heat stroke. They were in shock. My mother went to pieces, and my Dad was hollering, "No! No! No!" I tried to console my mother, and I did cry with her that evening. It hurt to see them hurting so much, besides finally realizing that I would never be able to talk to my brother again. Once they regained their composure, we started making plans to travel to Scottsdale. I told them that I would make the flight arrangements. I went home and called the airlines, made the arrangements, and then updated my parents.

It just happened that our daughter, Whitney, was on a summer trip to Tulsa, visiting friends and family. When we returned from my parents, Gwen had to call Whitney to make arrangements for her to get back home, so she could go with us. We were scheduled for a 10:00 a.m. flight on Monday morning. On Monday morning, I drove over to my parents' house, and we all rode to the airport together. Whitney flew into the airport from which we were leaving, so we were finally all together. Soon we learned that our flight was delayed for an unknown reason. We were originally scheduled to be in Phoenix by 4:00 in the afternoon, but we did not even leave San Antonio that day. Our flight was ultimately canceled, because of mechanical failures, and the airline put us up in a nearby hotel. They placed us on a 6:00 a.m. flight on Tuesday morning. Nothing was going right on this trip, and that was extremely hard on my parents. They were so anxious to get to Phoenix to console my sister-in-law and their grandchildren. We finally reached Phoenix on Tuesday morning.

A little side pressure in all of this was that I had only been working with my employer a little more than a year, and now I needed a week for bereavement. For the past six months, my employer had been so generous as I worked through the issues of the flooded house. Now this happens. Again, they were extremely considerate and generous to us. We will always remember that.

In the past, Gwen had expressed to me that she felt that if anything ever happened to me, she knew that she could turn to Gary as a source for providing her with sound guidance in what should be done. Now, his death was an even greater loss for her. We were all suffering.

My parents never overcame the loss of my brother. When June arrived each of the following years, they would schedule a trip to visit relatives out-of-state. They would stay away from home for two to three weeks, just before and just after June 27th. Anytime my mother thought about my brother, she began to cry. Based on many comments that my parents made to me, I know that they always mourned his death. He was their first child. He was very dear to them. My mother even made the comment that she knew there was a possibility that they would lose me, but never Gary. That was strictly based on the fact that I had battled cancer several times. At the same time, I believe that we should mourn for a time, and then move on. Since I have never suffered the loss of my own child, I can only talk about what I think I would do if I were to lose one of my children. I hope and pray that I will never experience that kind of loss. I frequently pray to God asking that I will never have to experience the death of one of my children. If I do, I pray that I will have the strength to accept the loss and continue on with my life in a meaningful way.

One message rang loud and clear to me, because of the death of my brother. You must always make the most of the time that you do have with loved ones, for life can be snatched away in a moment's notice. Do not leave anything unsaid between you and a loved one. Tell them how much you love them, appreciate them, and care for them. Take advantage of the opportunities that you do have. Do not assume that you will have many more opportunities later in life. Only God knows if you will.

Chapter 13

Struggles with My Parents

My parents created the following feelings for me. They were very loving, but also very possessive of my life. They expected me to bring my family to their house to visit them every weekend. Our schedule did not matter to them. I worked long hours during the week. I had to take care of the yard and other things on the weekend. I also played softball in the spring, summer and fall, plus basketball in the winter. Sports have always been very fulfilling to me in multiple ways. For one, they are a huge stress reliever. If I can go play an hour of basketball at lunchtime, I come back to work ready to tackle more things. My softball games were a family outing for us. We would all go to the game together. The boys would be batboys from time to time, plus they chased foul balls. Gwen sat and visited with the wives of the players, or kept score.

There are times when you just want to lounge around your own house on Sunday afternoon. My parents expected us to be at their house every Sunday. My mother would cook us lunch any time we said that we would be there to eat. If we missed a weekend, the next time we showed up at their house, there would be comments like, "Thought you had forgotten where we lived!" Besides everything else, Gwen and I always attended church on Sunday morning and Sunday evening. So we had to rush out to their house following church; take a change of clothes so that we could do things outside, then we had to dress again and leave for church that evening.

As our children got older, my dad would always keep a gentle horse around for the kids to ride. Some time after we would arrive at their house, my dad would disappear for a while, then the next thing we knew, he would be hollering for us to come outside. It was time for the kids to ride the horse. It was not a question of whether they wanted to ride, or not. It was time to ride. The other issue was, it was not just a casual ride. If the child did not hold the reins right, or make the horse go in the direction that my dad expected, he would yell at them. To them it was not fun. Horses were my dad's life. He always trained horses for polo. He expected everything to be done the right way. He was offended if the kids said they did not want to ride. And let me tell you, there was many a time when Gwen and I had to battle a crying child, to coerce them into riding the horse for Grandpa. If we did not, we knew that we would hear all of the negative comments from him later. You might be thinking that I should not have put up with that. You could be thinking that I should have had the guts to stand up to my father and tell him that my kids did not want to ride and not to expect us to be coming out to his house every weekend. I preferred to suffer through the situation and keep peace in the family.

Please hear me say this as well. My father did all of this out of love for us and for his grandchildren. That was the only way that he knew how to show his love. He was not a person with whom you could have a logical discussion and reason through these issues. That was not his nature. He had to be in control.

Another way in which my parents tried to control our lives involved visiting relatives. My dad in particular, had numerous relatives in Ohio and Kentucky. They were all great people, many of them I never knew, because my parents were not big on vacations when I was small. I can remember taking two trips to Ohio and Kentucky—one when I was 8, and one when I was 14. One other time, my mother and I traveled to Ohio when I was 18. Therefore, I was not very close to my relatives. When my children were old enough to start playing baseball in the summer, I was very involved in coaching their teams. It was about that time, that it seemed like a lot of those relatives began making trips to Oklahoma to visit my parents.

I want to emphasize that the following statements are not about my relatives. We did enjoy visiting with them. The point is my parents' attitude. They expected us to stop our lives. Our priorities were not important to them. They had no respect for us. Gwen or I would get a call a day or two before someone was going to be in town, asking us to come out and spend time with them, or, informing us that they were going to bring them out to our house. Many times, we would be eating supper and our doorbell would ring. My parents would just show up unannounced with relatives. The condition of our house did not matter to my parents, but it did to us. We did not have a chance to prepare the house. My parents would start giving the relatives or friends a tour of our house without asking. The downstairs was usually okay, but they would take them upstairs. The bedrooms were usually a mess, because that is where our children often played with their friends. Beds were often not made, or clothes were on the floor. With three active, young children and their friends being at our house, plus our family spending so much time at the baseball fields, our home could easily be in shambles when they showed up. In addition, we might be getting ready to go to a game within minutes. Their intentions were good, but they were not considerate of our feelings or schedule. My parents did not understand what it was like to have three children from the ages of six to ten, all participating in sports at the same time. They thought they did, because they had two sons, but it was totally different since we were born eight years apart. There were only one or two years when my parents had both of us playing sports at the same time. It appeared that they had forgotten about those times, plus my parents were never involved in coaching my teams. That took a lot of time on my part, but it also allowed me to spend quality time with my children. My parents even went so far as to enter our house when we were not home. We had provided them with a key as a backup, in case we lost ours, but since they had a key, they thought that it was okay to take friends and family to see our home while we were at work, without ever asking us.

I felt like I was treated as a possession, being their child, even when I was forty years old. Because of the expectations that they placed on my family, I made a very conscience decision that I would never treat my children or their families that same way. I had so much resentment toward my parents. It is my opinion that parents should not smother their children once they leave home. They should treat them as grown adults that have choices in life that must be honored. Second, parents should not attempt to keep a tight reign on their children once they have moved away. At that point, the children should be in control of their own lives.

Chapter 14

The Death of My Parents

My parents were all excited. One of their grandchildren was coming to visit. On June 21, 2002, my parents had taken my niece sightseeing. They came to our house that evening to celebrate my oldest son's birthday. We all had a great evening, visiting around the dinner table, and then continuing our visit afterwards. We took pictures with my niece and parents; my niece with our children and my niece with my family. While taking the pictures, the thought never entered our minds that this would be our last opportunity for photos of my mother while she was healthy. That is not something that you normally consider when everyone is together having a great time. My mother had been a very active person for her age and appeared to be very healthy. That evening the women were all sharing stories and laughing. That was a perfect night as far as my parents were concerned, because family meant everything to them.

About 8:30 that evening, my parents decided it was time to return to their house, and my niece went to stay with them. That same night, shortly after my mother went to bed, she suffered a massive brain hemorrhage, a stroke. My dad awoke to her trembling on her side of the bed, but she could not move or speak. My father yelled to my niece and she called 9-1-1. About 2:00 a.m., June 22, I was awakened by a phone call. My niece was calling from the hospital to inform us that my mother had suffered a stroke and they had called the ambulance to take her to the hospital. Gwen and I rushed to get dressed and headed to the hospital. We called Todd and Garrett. They came to the hospital in New Braunfels a short time later. Once my mother reached the hospital, the emergency room physician immediately called for a CT Scan. When Gwen and I arrived at the hospital, the physician met with the family and told us that my mother's prognosis was very bleak. He said there was a large mass in her brain that was creating tremendous pressure in her head. He further informed us that there was little hope for her recovery. She had a mass of blood about the size of a tennis ball in her brain. He did not see any hope for her, but my father pressed for him to contact another doctor. He found a neurosurgeon in San Antonio that reviewed the CT scans and was willing to do surgery. He provided some hope that my mother could return home at some point.

My mother was transported via ambulance to the San Antonio hospital about 6:00 a.m. Surgery did not start until late that afternoon, because of the doctor's busy schedule. After the surgery, her surgeon informed us that the blood clot was roughly the size of a tennis ball. It was considerably worse than he had anticipated. He informed us that only time would tell us what her outcome would be. He felt that she would regain some of her speech and would regain some mobility. My father clung to that hope. Her right side was paralyzed following the stroke, and she could not see out of her right eye. She never regained vision in her right eye. The next morning, my mother was able to speak a few words. Over the next month, she probably regained about five to ten percent of her vocabulary. The clot had damaged the brain in the area of speech. She could not do very simple things like count to three, or name a color that you held in front of her. She did have an understanding of who was in the room with her. It was very clear that she recognized immediate family.

Mother was in Intensive Care for ten days. When and if she improved, she would be moved to a regular, private room. During the doctor's next visit, he informed my father that we should move her to a rehabilitation hospital. He provided a list of facilities in the area. She was in a transplant hospital and that facility could not provide the appropriate rehabilitation. Gwen and I had our jobs that we had to be at during the days, so we were not a part of this discussion. Whitney was present, because she drove my father to the hospital. My dad was never a good communicator. He kept things to himself. It became apparent that my father was not going to ask anyone to help find another facility, and he was not checking it out either. Soon, Whitney started calling hospitals from the list that the doctor provided. She arranged two interviews, where a hospital counselor came and interviewed my father and viewed my mother. A quick decision had to be made, because the rehab hospital had a very limited number of beds. Gwen and I were not even aware of this situation until after it was done. My seventeen-year-old daughter "took the ball and ran with it." Thanks to Whitney, a very good rehabilitation facility accepted my mother. Had it not been for her hard work and making it happen, who knows where my mother would have been sent? It was later that the rehab facility realized that she was a granddaughter, only seventeen, and making all of the arrangements, or they may not have listened to her. They thought she was a daughter.

One of the many changes in my mother was that she became very vocal toward my father and his actions. She could only speak a few words, but those, coupled with her action, showed us that she was a very different person. My father had a hard time dealing with this change. He was very determined in his own way that he was going to will her back to health. He was totally devoted to her care. He would leave his house at sunrise, because he could not drive in the dark, and he would be at the hospital all day. Gwen and I would get

off work; meet at home and rush to the h
could leave and get back home before d
nurses tried to get my father to take d
but he felt that he was the only person w
mother the way she needed.

Because he was so controlling, that provoked a
mother's anger. He would watch her lying in bed; then
would get up and move her to where he thought she ought to
be. He would take a cool, wet washcloth and wash her face,
much more often than she wanted. He would tell me to do
things, and then mother would hear that and get angry at
what he said to me.

There was another dynamic that really frustrated my
father. When Gwen and I entered her hospital room in the
evening, she would see us and start smiling, and often greeted
us with, "Hi there!" or, "Oh, it is you." The problem was that
she was so frustrated with my father and was very hateful,
until Gwen and I walked into the door. When she saw us, it
was like we were there to rescue her and she began to smile
and talk. He would tell us that she had not been talking. It
would frustrate him when she would respond so positively to
us. The positive attention was not on him or for him. He was
not the one she looked to for comfort and that hurt him. He
could never understand that he was causing many of the
problems by being so overbearing with her. My father tried to
get my mother to tell him "I love you", but she would not.
However, she would tell Gwen and me "I love you" without
a problem. Before the stroke, Mother would tell my dad "I
love you" whenever he left the house to go somewhere.

I do not know how to convey just how awkward the
situation really was. My father thought that he knew better
than any of the doctors or nurses or family about how my
mother should be cared for. That was evident at the
rehabilitation hospital. Everyday that we entered her room,
all the window shades were closed; the television was turned

and she was lying in a softly lit room. Gwen and I had lgthy conversations with the nursing staff at the ehabilitation hospital. The nurses told us that my mother needed stimulation and encouraged us to bring items such as family photos, flowers, a radio and other things that might help to increase her vocabulary. In general, they expressed that she needed a bright, cheery room to keep her from being depressed. They had spoken to my father about this, but he would not listen. They came to us to try to get him to understand, but he would not listen to us either. When my father left for the evening, we would open the window shades and let her see out. She did not care to watch TV. I even tried to read Bible scriptures to her at times, but she could not focus for very long.

Dealing with my father during this time was very challenging, to put it diplomatically. First, he suffered from macular degeneration. He was legally blind, although he still argued that he could see well enough to drive. For the first two weeks, either my daughter or niece drove him to the hospital, but it came time for my niece to return home, and my daughter moved away for college. Keep in mind that Gwen and I had full-time jobs during all of this. One of his neighbors volunteered to drive him each day, but he refused to let him help. At that point, Gwen and I offered to drive him to the hospital each day. My dad insisted that he could drive himself. One of the doctors at the rehabilitation center had told my dad that there was a "back way" to the hospital from his house. We are talking forty-five miles, one way. That was not a short trip. I drove him to the hospital two times, on the exact same route, so that he could count the number of intersections that he would pass before his turn. Amazingly, he drove himself to the hospital without a wreck for three weeks. He could only drive in the daylight, but he made it. Gwen and I would drive up there each evening as soon as we got home from work to help watch my mother, so he could drive home before dark. Fortunately, this was during the summer months. I do not know what we would have done if this had been during the winter months when it gets dark by the time I get home.

Many days, my mother refused to go to rehabilitation. My father would argue with her, insisting that she had to go to get better. My father did not understand. In her mind, she did not want to deal with the strenuous exercise. She would get very frustrated with her inability to do things that were once no problem for her. It was too difficult. He knew that the only way she would ever be able to return home, would be if she would get strong enough to get up and get in a wheel chair and eat on her own. For weeks, she also refused to eat. The hospital staff kept her going through intravenous feedings. My father kept insisting that she eat. I can remember her reaching up and grabbing my father by the shirt and pulling him down to within inches of her face. Her facial expressions exhibited a fury within her. She screamed, "Johnny! I said NO!" Do you think that my father got the message? No way! He took it as a sign that she was still strong. He did not understand that he was extremely frustrating to her. He laughed when she got angry. My dad thought he was making her stronger by making her fight back. He was used to my mother almost always agreeing with him and going along with what he wanted. She was different now. If she did not want to do something, there was no way that he was going to make her do it.

Please, do not misunderstand me. My mother's love for my father was not gone. She still had a very strong love for him. When he was kind and gentle with her, they got along great. But, when he became too demanding, she was no longer going to put up with it. She was very vocal and demonstrative with her feelings. She had never been that way before. She was always very happy and willing to go along with my father's wishes. My mother did not have the same personality after the stroke that she possessed all of the previous years. For the first time in her married life, she was frequently confronting my father.

After thirty-five days at the rehab facility, it was determined that my mother was not improving at the pace that justified her staying in this facility versus a nursing home. She constantly refused rehab. Her rehabilitation was always scheduled during the day, when I had to be at work, so I do not know what the real issues were. My mother may have given up on ever being able to walk again. She may have been waging a war against my father, because he was being so forceful trying to get her to participate in the exercises. Her hospital Medicare benefit was being used up and the staff recommended that we move her to a nursing home, instead of wasting her hospital rehabilitation benefits that she refused to use. There is a limit on the number of days for which Medicare will pay for hospital services. To justify her continued stay, the hospital had to be able to report progress to Medicare for the continuance of benefits. Since she was refusing rehab, they could not justify keeping her there. After the hospital counselor delivered this message to my father, he tried to relay the message to me, but the details became very confusing. My father was hard of hearing and very troubled with my mother's condition; so that and many other factors added to the communication difficulties. I had to schedule a meeting with the counselor in order to understand the real issue. Once I spoke with the counselor, I was then able to explain to my father why it was necessary to move my mother. The hospital needed her moved quickly. The way my father talked, I thought that he was working with the counselor and talking with nursing homes. Then, one afternoon, he called and said, "Have you found a nursing home yet?" I had no clue that he needed us to look. He was the only person that could choose her facility. He was the spouse.

He had to sign the papers. His actions made us believe that he was handling it. Out of the blue, I received that phone call.

There was a maximum of one hundred days of continuous hospital care that would be covered by Medicare. She could be moved to a nursing home and be covered for an additional period of time, with two qualifications. She either had to be fed intravenously, or else she had to be showing progress in her rehabilitation. A counselor was assigned to my mother at the hospital, but they did not do a lot of research. It was important to Gwen and me that my mother be moved to a nursing home as close to home as possible. From June 21 until August 4, we were driving forty-five miles each way to visit and care for my mother, multiple times some days. According to the counselor, there were no empty beds in New Braunfels. They were recommending a nursing home in San Antonio to my father. Gwen started calling the homes in New Braunfels. It was very discouraging, because their response was that all of their beds were full, but if a bed became available, they would give us a call. She contacted one nursing home, and the lady was very compassionate about our situation. Fortunately, a room became available in New Braunfels and my mother was transported there. The home was only one and a half miles from my father's house, and the physical therapist was very good with my mother. What a relief for all of us!

The whole situation surrounding my mother's stroke made it very difficult to know what to do and what not to do. It appeared to me that my father wanted to be the decision maker in everything. He spoke to the surgeon and decided that the surgery should be performed to remove the clot. That was the right decision. But as weeks went by, he made comments to my daughter that I should be making some of the decisions that we faced. How was I to know? He never asked me for my opinion, but he expected me to do things. To say the least, it was a very frustrating situation. Looking back, we are certain that he was suffering from dementia. By law, the doctors could only act on his demands, because he was her spouse.

Toward the end of my mother's stay at the rehabilitation hospital, my father's best friend, Raymond, traveled from Tulsa to stay with him for a week. During that time, Raymond drove my father to the hospital and they visited my mother every day. There was a new dynamic emerging in all of this. My father's friend was a very happy-go-lucky type of person. He enjoyed life and joked a lot. I could see that my father was getting frustrated with Raymond, because he was joking around, trying to make the situation better. That did not help my father. It was similar to my father being frustrated when he saw that my mother was much happier when Gwen and I came to visit, than when he was there alone with her.

That friend relayed some frustrating information to me after my father's death. The information involved me taking care of the bills and writing checks. My father could not see well enough to write a check, therefore, with my mother in the hospital, he asked me to come over to his house twice a week to go through the mail and write checks for any bills that he received. I did just that. In addition, each time I was writing checks, he asked me if we needed any money. Each time I answered, "No thanks. We are doing fine." That was the truth and I never wrote myself a check. However, here is what the friend relayed to me. My father expressed a lot of frustration to the friend, because he just knew that I was stealing money from him. He never questioned me about it, but he was convinced that I was writing checks to myself. A simple review of the checkbook would prove that I had done nothing of the sort. This stemmed from the fact that I asked him to go to the bank and have my name and signature added to his banking account. Several of my friends recommended that I do this. If something happened to my father I would have access to my parents' bank account to care for my mother. Although my father had never had any problem with me stealing his money, or anything else from their house, he had this contrived notion that I had started taking from him. By my father's best friend relaying this problem to me, it helped me to better understand some of the things that my father voiced frustration with in the prior months. Raymond told my father that there was no way that Gene would do such a thing. He actually expressed it in more emphatic language.

After my mother was moved to the nursing home, Gwen spent hours at home copying family photos and creating a collage of family photos for my mother. She had already decorated her room with flowers and bright items, making it very cheerful. She did this with hope that my mother would be reminded of things from the past and her brain would be stimulated. Again, the nurses and doctors that we spoke to insisted that my mother needed pictures and other reminders. We were trying to do what we understood to be best for my mother. One Sunday afternoon, Gwen and I went to visit my mother with the finished collage. My mother sat up in bed. As Gwen pointed to pictures and made comments, my mother was shaking her head and laughing about things. There were a few times when tears came to her eyes as we discussed the grandchildren. She missed them. It was clear that my mother was enjoying the collage. My father called me out to the hallway, outside of my mother's room. His face was beet red. He was furious and proceeded to tell me that he did not want us discussing church stuff with my mother any more. Further, he demanded that we remove the photos on the wall. He believed that it only made her sad, yet all of the nurses kept encouraging us to bring pictures and other things that would remind her of things that she loved to do. I stood up to my father that day. He also told me that I needed to spend more time at the nursing home with my mother. I informed him that was not possible. I had only missed two days in the last three weeks, and that was because I had things to do at work and at home. I told him that Gwen and I were doing everything that we could to make her as happy and as comfortable as possible. Mother was really enjoying the personal attention from Gwen. After all, she had never experienced the love and care from a daughter…combing her hair, or rubbing her feet and hands with lotion — girl's stuff. My father resented it. Everything that we were doing was done because we were trying to help and we wanted to be there. I informed him that I could not do anymore than what I was doing and there was no way that I would ever be able to make him happy. This had been an overriding issue for years. Gwen and I could never visit enough to meet their expectations. I never was able to be at their house as often as he expected us.

My mother's ordeal finally became too difficult for my father to deal with. The doctors had made it clear that she would never be able to return home. On August 31, he committed suicide. I never saw this coming. I never suspected him committing suicide. It was different for Gwen though. She had discussed this very topic with her sister, and our daughter. The tendencies that she saw in my father indicated to her that he was a prime candidate to take his life. She had gone so far as to call my mother's doctor, but a call was never returned. She was obviously right. On Saturday morning, August 31, 2002, Gwen and I awoke and went to breakfast. Our lives had just entered a new phase — the empty nest syndrome. Our daughter had moved into her apartment at college, my middle son had moved back to college, so this was the beginning of our first school year without children living at home. After breakfast, we went to the high school and watched a volleyball game, then we drove to San Antonio to do some shopping. This was our first "free time" in months, with work, with my mother's stroke, and then my daughter moving off to college. That afternoon we made sure that we arrived at the nursing home in time to feed Mother her dinner, and get her ready for bed. That would allow my father time to go home early and relax. When we arrived at the nursing home and entered my mother's room, it was odd that my father was not there. We suspected that he had gone down to the kitchen area with my mother's roommate. He did that at times. My mother was sobbing when we entered her room, but we did not know why. Since she could not communicate very well, we could only speculate about what caused her to be so sad. Her dinner tray arrived and I started feeding her. While I was doing that, Gwen went down to the kitchen. She saw my mother's roommate and asked her if she had seen my father during the day. With a puzzled look, she told her, "No, he has not been here all day" and she was concerned. This lady always looked forward to seeing my father. He brought her the morning paper, candy and mints. It was not like him, because he was always there, or he told them specifically when he would be there. So Gwen came back to my mother's room, while I was feeding her, and told me that my father had not been there all day. My response was, "There's nothing that we can do now. Let me finish feeding Mother and we can go over to his house." Gwen was surprised by that response, but in my mind, I expected to find my father dead of a heart attack at home. If he had not been at the nursing home that day, I knew that death was the only thing that would keep him away. When I finished feeding my mother and got her settled for the evening, Gwen and I left and headed towards my parents' house. It was less than two miles away. In the car we were both silent at first, but then I told Gwen, "I expect to find my father dead." She was shocked and said, "Oh Gene! No!" She did not want me thinking that, but I told her that is the only thing that would keep my father from being with my mother at the nursing home. I did not realize that Gwen was thinking the same thing. When we arrived at his home, it was still daylight outside, but the house was dark, with no lights on inside. His car was under the carport, so it appeared that he had not gone anywhere. I unlocked the back door, opened it and hollered for my father. There was no answer. I stepped inside, and started turning on lights, but it was such an eerie feeling—I thought I might find him lying dead, but at the same time, I did not know exactly what to expect. I slowly walked through the kitchen, then through the living room, continuing to call out for my father. There was still no sign of him. I went to his bedroom, then bathroom, but nothing. He was not in the house. Gwen and I met in the dining room. We looked down on the table and there was a note, written in pencil, with large letters. It was a struggle to make out the words, but when we did, there was no doubt what it meant. We both rushed outside. She looked in the front yard, then headed across the street to speak with one of the neighbors. I went into the back yard. It was dusk, so you could not see very well. My father was not in the backyard, but then I walked over to the fence around the small garden area. There I saw his body with his face to the ground. I spoke, "Daddy? Daddy?" There was no response. I saw a blanket wrapped around his right arm and I knew that he was dead, so I went to the front of the house and yelled to Gwen that I had found him. As we ran into the back yard, she told me to stay back and she entered the garden. She did not want me to see him in that horrible condition. She told me that he had shot himself, which I was certain of by then. We then called 9-1-1 to report a suicide. Within fifteen minutes, the first police car arrived. We met the policeman at the front of the house and told him how we had found my father. During the conversation, to some degree, it became apparent that we were being questioned as suspects. That was a little scary in itself. Police dispatched the director of a funeral home to remove his body. That took about one and one-half hours. While the police were still there, we were standing outside on the front lawn.

The neighbors started coming over to see what was going on. Gwen and I were very concerned about how the neighbors would react to us. What kind of stories had my dad told them about us? It was soon apparent that they had heard the stories, but they did not believe my father. All of the neighbors were very comforting to us. They offered assistance with arrangements or help with my mother or whatever we needed. One of them specifically mentioned a few stories my dad had told him, but he went on to say that he had met me before and knew that was not the real situation. That small group of neighbors continued to support us until we sold the house. They kept an eye on the place and that was a huge relief.

I honestly believe that one of the contributing factors to my father's suicide was that he no longer had control over me, or of my mother. If he did not have control, he did not know how to live. It is a true shame when a person reaches that point in his or her life.

My father's suicide note read:

I cannot lift her any more. I cannot see. I love her.

That showed his focus. He could only think of his weaknesses and my mother. He never offered any apology to me for wanting to end his life, or asked for my forgiveness. He never wrote, "I love you" to me or to any of his grandchildren. It was all about him and my mother. She was his "eyes', his caregiver and he loved her with all of his heart.

I learned that some people are never satisfied. They choose to always look at life in a negative way. Instead of asking, "What has someone done for me today?" and show appreciation, instead they ask, "What has someone not done for me today?" To use an old cliché, they look at the glass of water as half empty, not half full. My father was not willing to look for ways to be happy without my mother. He did not recognize how much the rest of us cared about him. Gwen and I have discussed this with a lot of people and we do not believe that our parents ever thought that we would be as devoted to them in a time of need as we were. Gwen did not miss a day of going to the nursing home to visit my mother. She worked nearby and would visit Mother more than once a day—before work, during lunch and after work. On my way from work, I brought dinner for us and we would spend the entire evening in her room. I would visit at least six days a week, and many times seven days. We are comfortable with the way that we conducted ourselves during that trying time, even though my father expressed to me that I should have been visiting more. In my mind, I did everything that I could. My normal life was totally ignored. All of the regular pleasures in our life were put on the shelf for five months. That is all you can do. I encourage everyone to react in a similar way. Do all you can to help, and then you will never regret not having done enough.

I was the only remaining child. My mother's care was now in my hands. She could no longer read or write, but she could understand most of what I told her. Months earlier I was visiting my parents one day and during our conversation, my mother said, "We have something that we want to discuss with you and Gwen. We have decided that we want to be cremated when we die. We do not want any big ceremony or costly funeral. We want it to be simple." In fact what my mother used to tell me was, "When I get old and senile, just put me in a nursing home and forget about me. I do not want to be any trouble for you. When I die, just put me in a pine box and bury me." That was her message. Then they changed it a little bit and asked if cremation was okay with us. We assured them that it was. Now, with the death of my father, and my mother unable to communicate her wishes, I told the funeral home director to cremate my father's remains. He asked if my mother was still alive. I told him, "Yes, but she cannot communicate any more." He then asked, "Do you have Power of Attorney for your mother?" Unfortunately I did not. Therefore, I could not direct him to cremate my father without my mother's written consent. This all occurred the same evening that I found my father dead. What was I to do? The problem was compounded by the fact that my father did not leave a Will. Days earlier, he told me that he had attempted to make an appointment with a friend that had offered to write a Will for him, but they could not get together. On a couple of occasions, I had asked him to have a Will prepared, so he made the contact, but did not follow through.

There was no way that I was going to the nursing home at 10:00 p.m. and tell my mother of my father's death. I had the responsibility once before when my brother died, and I could not bare to tell my mother of her great loss a second time.

Delivering the News to my Mother

The following morning, I called my mother's doctor. I explained the situation and asked if she would meet me at the nursing home and explain to my mother what had happened. I had no idea how my mother would respond to the news of my father's death, so there was no way that I wanted to deliver that message to her without the doctor present. The doctor and I agreed to meet at the nursing home around noon. We met in the lobby and discussed the details of the situation. We came to the agreement that the doctor would deliver the news to my mother. I hoped that she would be able to tell my mother in a way that would be less painful than if I were to tell her, partially because she was a female and females tend to be more compassionate in times like this. One of my problems has always been that I am a person of few words. I get right to the point too quickly.

When we entered the room, my mother was sobbing. That was the same way that Gwen and I found her on Saturday evening. The doctor and I sat down on the bed with her and began to speak with her. My mother's doctor did a wonderful job of informing her of my father's death. We had agreed that we would only tell her that his heart quit beating. Mother cried for a few minutes, then she seemed to feel better. It is only speculation, but we believe that my father had told her "good bye" on Friday evening. I believe that my mother was grieving my father's departure. I am not certain just what he told her, but she was definitely missing my father. I asked her if she was and she said yes.

As the doctor left, I asked her if she would write a letter to confirm that my mother was of sound mind. The doctor expressed her confidence in my mother's ability to understand what she was being told. I needed the letter to take to my attorney so that a Will could be drawn up and my mother could inform them that my father was to be cremated. That was all completed by Wednesday of the same week.

Once my mother was informed, the next difficult task was to inform all of my father's family and friends of his death. My father still had two living sisters, plus numerous relatives and friends. It took two and one-half days to contact everyone. Of course, everyone was asking when the funeral would be held. I was not certain. I really struggled with this decision. My parents had only lived in New Braunfels for two years. They did not have many local friends since they were new to the area. Most of my father's relatives did not travel anymore, so they would not be able to attend the funeral service. My mother was not able to attend, so we decided not to have one. That was not a popular decision with some family members and friends. Although no one said they believed that I should have a service, I did, on multiple occasions, have several family members ask if we had already had the services. I knew that my parents did not expect, nor desire, a large ceremony. More than once, they told me, "Just put me in a pine box and bury me." I discussed the funeral situation with all of the grandchildren, most of whom were attending colleges in several different locations. They stated that they were busy with school and work. We all agreed that a funeral ceremony was not necessary. Further, the present time was not a convenient time for everyone to come together. I would have arranged a service if they needed it, but they assured me that they did not. I specifically requested that they notify me in advance when they would be free to gather and have a memorial service.

We were also dealing with several different emotions. My children were angry at my father for abandoning me when my mother needed so much care. They could not understand why he would be so selfish and only think about his loss. I understood those emotions, but I tried to explain to my children why they should not be angry with him. I too was shocked at what he had done, but I knew that he had been unstable in his thinking in recent weeks. He was totally lost and in great pain. The love of his life was struggling to live and her quality of life was gone. He could not stand to see her in that condition, nor could he imagine life without her.

I could not imagine that my father would want us to celebrate him taking his own life. I do not understand how anyone could be proud of such an act. Not celebrating his life was the right decision for me. I had always been taught that you honor someone while they are alive. The funeral ceremonies are for those still living and that is my belief. My decision was best for our immediate family. I hope that my relatives have grown to understand and accept that decision. I discussed my decision to not have a ceremony with several of my parents' closest friends and they now understood my decision. It was a decision that was made after I received input from many others, and one that I struggled with for several days. My initial impression was to not have a ceremony, but I considered the feelings of others who were close to my parents.

After my mother passed, Gwen and I made an appointment with the Veteran's Burial Director at the Sam Houston National Cemetery for veterans in San Antonio, Texas. Arrangements were made for my parents to be interred there. My father was proud of his military service in World War II. He remained close to several men in his immediate company, particularly his Lieutenant, whom he credited for keeping him alive during his thirty months overseas. Having him buried in a national cemetery would have been an honor to him. His and my mother's remains lie there together. I am confident that they would be pleased with that choice.

Choosing to Stop Food For My Mother

One of the toughest decisions that I have ever been faced with concerned my mother's life. On my list of "hardest things I have ever done in my life", it ranks right up there with having to inform my parents that my brother had died. I do not know which task was more difficult. I truly empathize with anyone who is faced with those situations. There was nothing easy in either of those tasks. My mother was a healthy, seventy-nine-year-old, who got around without a problem, until she suddenly suffered a stroke.

We were advised that it would be best to stop her food intake, but we had to make the final decision. That tough decision was required when my mother suffered a second stroke at the nursing home. The stroke caused her to lose more of her abilities. What little vocabulary she had before, was now gone. She was frequently sobbing when we entered her room. The brain damage was severe in the part of her brain that controlled emotions. When I tried to feed her, she could not focus on the food, nor her chewing of the food. She began to constantly drool as she ate, which she had never done in the past. Soon, she refused to eat and intravenous feedings began. When her condition continued to worsen, the counselor at the nursing home informed us that it was probably time to call Hospice. Hospice was contacted and we were very fortunate to have a wonderful local Hospice organization. They moved very quickly to help us. A Hospice nurse visited my mother three times a week to care for her. They provided a better wheelchair than was currently available at the nursing home. In October, the nurse met with us to discuss what was best for my mother. My mother was not responding to anyone. Her ability to speak was gone. She did not desire food. She merely existed. The life that she had enjoyed was gone. The Hospice nurse said that her kidneys were not functioning normally, and that it would actually be less painful for my mother if we did not feed her. She explained that giving my mother the intravenous feedings would only prolong her agony and would cause swelling of her body and pain. In the nurse's estimation, there was no hope for recovery. It was very likely that my mother was continuing to suffer small strokes, leading up to another massive one. With that information, the final decision was left to Gwen and to me. A lot of questions run through your head at that point. Am I doing this in my mother's best interest or for myself? Am I being selfish? What will be going through my mother's mind? Will she realize that we are not feeding her? Will she thank us for this or will she be thinking that we want her to die?

I prayed to God that I would make the right decision. Gwen and I discussed our options. We reviewed what each of us had heard from the Hospice staff and from the nursing home staff. After a lot of prayer, thought and discussion, Gwen and I decided that the right thing to do was to stop giving her food. She would only receive medications to comfort her. We had to rely on the expertise of the Hospice nurse. She had seen many similar situations. Our conclusion was that she obviously knew what was best for a person in my mother's condition. The nurse had told us that she would probably live from three days to three weeks. My mother continued to live without food for twenty-one days. It was hard to understand how she could continue to live that long. During the final week, she was barely coherent. The medications had her "knocked out" for the most part. She was resting in comfort and that was most important to us. We continued to visit her every evening. On the final night, she had a great deal of difficulty breathing. I sat beside her and talked to her although her eyes were closed. I prayed aloud on her behalf. Gwen was also there providing comfort. I told Mother that I loved her and that she was going to a better place, to Heaven. At 8:30 p.m., I hugged her, then kissed her goodbye and told her that I loved her again. Her breathing was very shallow and labored, but she did not appear to be suffering. Her eyes told me that she was ready to leave this world. At about 10:30 p.m. that evening, the nursing home called us and told us that mother had passed away. They asked if we wanted to come be with her, but that was not necessary for us. We had been by her side, almost every day for the past five months. I was glad that she was no longer suffering. I believe that she had gone to a better place, to Paradise, and our prayers had been answered.

Chapter 15

Lessons Learned During Life-Altering Events

When you face a crisis any number of reactions is possible. You may be overcome with deep depression. Your first impulse may be to deny that it is real. Running from the situation may be a temptation. Or, you may choose to confront the issue head-on and make the best of a bad situation. I know that is easier said than done, but I can also guarantee you that it is possible to confront and conquer. Go one step further by searching for lessons to be learned by confronting the situation. Those lessons learned will make you stronger when faced with another calamity. Here are some suggestions from my lessons learned, based on some of the crises with which we have dealt.

The First Cancer Diagnosis

My first indication that I could have a health problem came when I noticed the lump in my neck while I was shaving. I could have ignored that lump. I could have said, "It is no big deal. I am young and healthy. It is nothing!" But, I did not. I did think that it was probably just allergies that were causing my glands to swell, because I had moved to a new area, with many more cedar trees than I was used to. Gwen and the kids were having a lot of allergy problems themselves. I took a decongestant and the lump appeared to get smaller for a while, but it never went away.

When anyone mentions to me that something is not quite right with the way they feel, I strongly encourage them to "listen to their body!" What are your symptoms telling you? Do not deny that something is wrong. Do not be afraid to go to the doctor, because you are afraid that you might receive bad news. If there is bad news to be received, you need to hear it sooner rather than later. The earlier a disease is detected, the better your chances for successful treatment. Worse case is, you learn that you have a terminal illness or a disease that will cause you to be handicapped. Learning that early will give you more time to prepare for bad times ahead, when your capabilities will be lessened. Also, when I'm telling a young person about my story of cancer, I try to emphasize the importance of never ignoring signs that something could be wrong. Denial will only lead to disappointment and grief if there really is a health problem.

A second lesson learned dealt with how the diagnosis was presented. The doctor was very direct and to the point. That was the only way he knew to deliver such a bleak message. He was a very caring individual. He said, "You've got cancer, Hodgkin's disease. The biopsy has been sent for a second opinion, but the doctors are confident in the diagnosis." If you receive what appears to be a very harsh, thoughtless message, delivered with no care, do not judge the doctor to be a cold, unconcerned individual. If the doctor or nurse is very blunt, or appears "cold", when they are discussing test results, do not assume that they do not care and are just callused about the whole situation. Delivering the news could be very difficult for them, particularly if they happen to be the same age as you. After our meeting with my surgeon, the receptionist said she knew it was not good news because the surgeon had been pacing the floor since receiving and reading my pathology report prior to our visit. There was no doubt in my mind that he cared a great deal. He did not know a better way to deliver the bad news, except to get right to the point. There was no other way, in his mind, to deliver the bad news.

My first diagnosis of cancer and the resulting regimen of treatments changed another aspect of my life. Remembering to take pills at the prescribed times used to be very difficult for me. First, I did not like taking medications. Second, I was not ill very often, so I never formed a habit of being on a medication schedule. Prior to cancer, I was horrible when it came to remembering that I needed to take a pill, but that changed with my diagnosis of cancer. I was focused on doing everything exactly as the doctor prescribed. Forming a habit and staying on schedule was not a problem for me any longer. Part of my treatments included taking Prednizone for ten days at a time. My doctor explained that Prednizone is lethal to lymphoma, but it can also make you a very different person. He warned us to watch for a personality change, such as becoming less patient or mean-tempered. If that occurred, other drugs could be tried. My personality did change at times. While on the Prednizone, my patience became very short. I remember one night in particular, when one of my sons had done something of which Gwen and I did not approve, I lost my composure! I started cursing and ranting, and that just was not the typical me. Once I realized what I had done, I broke down and cried. Gwen consoled me by telling me my reaction was due to the drugs. She understood that was not a typical reaction. I had three kids crying with their faces buried in pillows. When I realized that, I went to each of them, apologized for my actions and tried to comfort them. I truly regretted that event after it happened. My family had never heard words like that out of my mouth. There were several other situations where I was very short and harsh with my family, but that particular situation was the worst.

A great benefit from the new found focus was that my loved ones received comfort in knowing that I was diligent about taking my medications. That is a big deal for your spouse or your parents. Otherwise, they can become very discouraged when they get the impression that "you do not care enough to take care of yourself." That makes them worry more because they love you and are concerned for you, plus they want you to do everything the doctor prescribes so you will win the battle.

Dealing with chemotherapy treatments is not easy. The first treatment can be very unnerving, because the oncologist explains to you all of the possible side affects that you may experience as a result of the drugs being used. One drug can cause heart damage. Another may cause you to lose your hair, experience nausea, anxiety, and other negative side effects. Then you may be told that fourteen days after the treatment, your white blood count will drop drastically and you will be highly susceptible to any contagious infections or viruses. In fact, the oncologist explained that as a result of the chemotherapy, expect to be hospitalized two or three times in the six-month period. It is all so new to you. It is overwhelming. You will probably experience huge anxiety just during the first consultation regarding potential treatment. I have heard of numerous horror stories about people who had become deathly ill from chemotherapy. I am sure that you have too. That is scary in itself! Just remember that they need to prepare you, up front, for the worst-case scenario. It does not mean that you will definitely experience every one of these problems, but it is possible that you will.

Last, I do want to emphasize that overwhelming concern that overcame me after learning of my cancer—"the life insurance that I had never purchased" statement. In the past, I was not an advocate of insurance. My concern was that you could become "insurance poor," because there are so many different types of insurances that you do not necessarily need.

Plus, with three small children and owning a house, there was never any extra money for life insurance. When I was young and healthy, it seemed that I would be wasting money on life insurance premiums. Being the victim of a serious disease such as cancer can quickly change your opinion about insurance. You cannot afford to be without it. For example, health insurance is a must for any person employed full-time. Personal bankruptcy is a real possibility if you do not have healthcare insurance coverage and you are stricken with a serious disease, heart problems or other illnesses that require laboratory tests, doctor's visits and hospitalization. If you are the main provider for a family, do not try to save a few dollars by not paying health insurance premiums. Search for other ways to save money. One lengthy hospital stay without health insurance could become a financial nightmare.

Young folks, yes, you young people who are single or recently married, I know that you often believe "Nothing's going to happen to me! I do not need life insurance at this time in my life! I've got years before I need to worry about that. I need the money for a lot more important things than paying life insurance premiums." However, there comes a time in your life when life insurance does become vitally important. To me that was when I was diagnosed with cancer; I had three children, one in elementary, and two in middle school. Those children would one day need to go to college, and there was no way that my wife could afford to take on the family expenses, much less college expenses with her salary. You begin to think about those "bad decisions to not buy life insurance" when all of a sudden you realize that now you could not buy life insurance if you wanted to. Once you are diagnosed with cancer, you must be in remission for three to five years before the premiums are once again reasonable for someone with an average income. Each of you has to make the risk assessment for your own family. You may really be so financially strapped that there is no way for you to pay an insurance premium. I am not saying that you need to go into debt just to have it. I do want to encourage you to consider those loved ones that depend on your paycheck. If you are a single person, there may be no need to purchase a policy in your present situation. However, if you have a family or your plans are to have a family in the future, purchasing life insurance is something that you need to consider while you are healthy. If your health changed for the worse, you are stuck without a chance to purchase any. If the circumstance arises where you, or a member of your family, notices a lump or cyst somewhere on his or her body, and there is any possibility that surgery will be required to determine the seriousness of the cyst, and you do not have life insurance, I strongly urge you to purchase a life insurance policy prior to any surgery. You can always cancel the policy if the premium becomes a financial burden, or the test results come back negative. However, if the test results confirm that you have a disease, your opportunity to purchase that policy is gone, at least for the next five years. Each situation is different, but anytime you suspect that there might be a poor health situation, you better try to get an insurance policy before the diagnosis, if you know that you are not adequately insured or financially secure.

The Flood

You can never have too many friends. We often take our friendships for granted. Until you are going through difficult times, you don't realize how valuable they are. For the first two weeks after the flood, we lived with a family, because we did not have insurance that would pay for a hotel. We were greeted with open arms. The house was crowded with two families there, but our friends never complained. Their house was our house.

Another family offered us the use of their extra apartment that they had on their ranch. They said that we could stay there as long as needed. It was wonderful to have a place of our own again, where we didn't feel like intruders. We still had the monthly mortgage on our flooded house. That took all we had and we could not even live in that house. By July 1999, or about nine months later, we were finally able to move back into our home. Nine months—the use of the apartment was a huge gift.

Document Everything When A Disaster Occurs

Let me explain one of the important lessons learned from working through the aftermath of the flood. The details were mentioned earlier, but I will reiterate them here for emphasis. It was not just a little flooding. We had seventeen feet of water standing in our house for several hours. Our major problem was that we did not have any flood insurance. When we closed on our mortgage, it was not required. Another dynamic that caused anxiety was that I had a great deal of concern about my job, because I started that job only six months earlier. The flood occurred on Saturday. We worked cleaning the house and belongings all day Sunday. Come Monday, I had to call my boss to inform him of my flooded home and that there was no way I could be at work for several days. My employer was tremendous. They not only gave me the week off, but they sent people to help me clean up. My boss and his wife, came to our house, took a truckload of clothing home and washed it all for us. I soon realized just how lucky I was to be working for such a generous manager and such a great company. They even allowed another co-worker to take time off from work to help us. It took ten long days, working long hours, to clean out the house. Thank God that I worked for such a great company and we had so many gracious friends helping us on weekends.

When we originally attended the closing of our house purchase, the title company representative told us that no flood insurance was required. In looking at the closing papers that we uncovered following the flood, I discovered that our "Flood Determination" declaration stated that our property "...lies outside the 100-year flood plain." Our mortgage company did not require us to purchase flood insurance because of that document. If a piece of property lies inside the flood plain, a lending institution will require that you purchase flood insurance to protect their loan. Because we had been told that no flood insurance was necessary, we had always assumed that our house was not in danger of any flood. If we had known that the house was in a flood plain at the time of the purchase, it is highly unlikely that we would have ever purchased a home in that area.

Here is something else that we discovered. Flood insurance is not expensive when you have a mortgage on your house. For a house that later appraised at $200,000, the cost of the flood insurance was approximately $400 annually. I had always heard people talk about how expensive flood insurance was. Some families, who owned their house outright, told us that their flood insurance premium for a similarly valued house was in the range of $10,000 annually, because they did not have a mortgage. The flood insurance appears to be much less expensive, if you are paying a mortgage on the property insured by the flood insurance policy.

Now back to my suggestion. When your loss is due to a mistake on the part of a business, there are a few critical things you must do when contacting them. Here's what you need to do.

1. Before you call, get a notebook or planner so you can take notes of each conversation.

- Use the same notebook or planner every time you place a call to that institution.
- Be sure that you get the name of the person to whom you are speaking.

- Record the person's name and the date and time of the conversation.
- Your journal (notebook) should be a summary of every communication that you had with that organization, whether it was a phone call, e-mail, letter or hallway conversation.
- Take notes throughout the conversation in order to recall the details at another time.

2. Calling the organization

- As listed above, ask for the person's name
- Be cordial when you call. Do not lose your temper! Be calm, but firm. Be direct, but not defensive.
- Remember: **The people in customer service are NOT your problem!** They have to answer calls all day long from people who are often frustrated and vent to them.
- You may gain an advantage if you say something like, "I know that my problem is not with you, but I need your help." Explain your problem, and then ask, "Can you give me the name of the person responsible for <whatever product or service you are calling about>?"

3. Make notes of the conversation. What did you tell them? What was their response?

4. In the same notebook or planner, document the same details for each phone call.

5. When you write a letter, mention the date of the contacts, the name of the persons to whom you spoke and the context of the conversation.

- Keep a signed copy of every letter or email sent
- Make a folder; print or copy each document, then file it

- Do not depend on electronic documents saved on your computer, unless you make frequent backups of those documents—the day you need the copies is the day that your hard drive crashes, if you do not have a backup
- You should even note that you sent a communication in your planner or notebook, date, time, media used, etc.

HEAR ME ON THIS ONE! Do not wait until you have a major communication problem with this business or government office to start documenting your calls. START WITH THE FIRST COMMUNCATION! When you have any issue that may result in a major problem, start by documenting your first communication with them. This applies to billing problems that you are having with your wireless telephone carrier, to the set of custom golf clubs that you ordered over the Internet that need to be adjusted, to the transmission repair on your car, to the car wreck that you had recently and the other person was totally at fault, and to many other situations that could result in significant financial losses for you.

There is no doubt that proper documentation will cost you more of your personal time! That car repair is completed with no issues, or that billing error is corrected with the first call most of the time. But, when a major problem does arise, and you have documented every communication with that business or government office related to that major problem, you will be miles ahead. When you present that documentation to their top management, more than likely they will respond to you and correct the problem. If they do not respond, that documentation will help you in a small claims court.

I recovered over $150,000 during the flooded house situation, because of my detailed documentation, and persistence. It did not happen over night. It took from October 1998 until August 1999 before I had the final settlement check, but I did it without attorney fees. I was never rude, nor discourteous to the people on the other end of the phone. I was very persistent, quoting dates, times and names of persons to whom I spoke. I wrote sixteen letters to the mortgage company in a four-month period, finally getting to the right person. My letters were very factual, and I had a very helpful brother, who reviewed each letter before I sent it to the mortgage company. I would recommend that you find yourself someone who is business-minded that is willing to review your letters or emails prior to submitting them.

The better your documentation on each call, the better your case. If you ever had to get an attorney involved, your documentation would be tremendous evidence. Organized detail will convince others that you are telling the truth and it proves that you were diligent in working through the issue.

My Cancer Recurred Following the Flood

The flood occurred in October, and then in December I had an annual CT scan. The scan results showed that my cancer had returned only in my neck area. It was a horrible time for that kind of news. We were dealing with so many things, because of the flood. We could not live in our house, but we had the mortgage payment. How were we going to pay for our home to be rebuilt? At that time, the mortgage company was not being responsive to our needs. Gwen lost her part-time job, because of the flood. Now this.

The clear lesson in all of this was that cancer does not wait for a convenient time, and I could not ignore the diagnosis. Life's trials, disasters or diseases do not wait for a convenient time. In many cases, they will happen at the most troublesome time in your life. Your stress is compounded with the additional pressures, but you can get through those stressful times with the help of God, friends and family.

This was the third occurrence for the cancer to appear, so the news was not as shocking as previous times. Only twenty-one months had passed since the last episode, so that short time between my cancer recurring was somewhat discouraging. We did not know how many times my body could receive treatment before it would be too much to survive. After the initial treatments, I was in remission for four years, but this time, was after only twenty-one months. It felt like the cancer was becoming more difficult to treat. In my mind I questioned if it was a losing battle that I was fighting. Those negative thoughts only lasted a day or two, before I was prepared to fight again. Gwen and I had a strong faith that I would beat the cancer. We felt good that it only appeared in the neck area this time, and we hoped that radiation would possibly stop the cancer. Unfortunately, the cancer appeared on the opposite side of my neck eleven months later.

Death of My Parents

Lessen the burden for your children by preparing a Will before you die. Do not put off the task of preparing a Will, because you do not want to face the reality of it all. Soon after my first diagnosis of cancer, Gwen and I had one prepared. Unfortunately, my parents did not, but after my father's death, my mother's doctor visited with her, then wrote a letter concluding that she was cognizant and understanding of her surroundings. With that letter, I was able to go to an attorney, who drafted a Will, then sent assistants to the nursing home to review it with my mother and get her signature, or mark as it was at that time.

I learned that you cannot plan for the future with certainty. On multiple occasions, my parents told me how everything was prepared for my mother after my father passed. They were certain that my father would die first, then my mother. He did die first, but not as they intended. They expected him to die of natural causes first, because he was four years older than my mother. My father told me the car that he purchased in 2001 was the last car that my mother would need. Again, they were right, but he believed that she would be driving it after he died. My mother appeared to be in much better health than my father. His sight was failing him. His cholesterol level was always high. He had surgery twice to clean his corroded arteries. Mother's stroke came suddenly. My father went into shock when his plans were foiled. This reaffirmed to me the fact that you cannot plan death, unless you take it into your own hands, which is contrary to God's word. We do not have the right to take our lives or that of anyone else. We must always prepare ourselves spiritually for physical death. Only God knows when will be the judgment day. This is confirmed in **II Peter 3:10 (KJV)**.

> **II Peter 3:10** But the day of the Lord will come as a thief in the night; in the which the heavens shall pass away with a great noise, and the elements shall melt with fervent heat, the earth also and the works that are therein shall be burned up.

In **Romans 14:11, 12 (KJV)**, it teaches that each person is responsible for his own actions, not the actions of others.

> **Rom. 14:11** For it is written: "As I live, says the LORD, Every knee shall bow to Me, And every tongue shall confess to God."
> 12 So then each of us shall give account of himself to God.

Chapter 16

No Regrets

When I received the sudden news that my brother had died in 1999, or when I found my father dead in his garden of a self-inflicted gunshot wound, I had a lot of emotions running through my head. If I had failed to express my feelings to them prior to that time, it would have only compounded the matter. I can honestly say that I had no regrets regarding "unsaid words or love never expressed" when my brother died, or when my father died. I had voiced my love to my brother. While he was alive, we exchanged emails several times a week. In almost every email, we would end it with, "I love you." He was a tremendous help to me as I worked through the issues with the flood. He was my only brother, a friend and my financial advisor. He possessed a great deal of wisdom in the financial world, because he was a CPA and had been the CFO (Chief Financial Officer) of several companies. At the same time, he expressed a lot of love and support toward my family. He offered financial assistance when we were flooded. During my early years of marriage, he had several good, used cars to sell. He would always offer them to me first, of course, at a good price. During our last visit with him, he actually gave my oldest son a car. Granted, it was a twelve-year-old car, with over 100,000 miles, but it was still a good car. We have a picture of Todd and Gary in which Todd was giving him a one-dollar bill as payment. That was the last photo we took of my brother. All of those examples are stated, just to show a portion of how he demonstrated his love toward me.

With my father, there was a very different situation. My father was a hard-working person who always had to be in control. As I describe the situation in detail, I do not mean to paint a bad picture of my father. He loved our family and expressed that love in his own unique ways. It was the only way he knew how to express his love. He tried to do everything he could to make me successful in life. He just had a unique way of doing it. Everything had to be done his way to be pleasing to him. He was not flexible. About two years prior to his death, during some counseling sessions, I came to the realization that a lot of my personal success was due to my father never acknowledging my accomplishments when I was young. He was always willing to critique my efforts in sports, or my chores at home. In his eyes, things could have always been done better. Because of his attitude, I worked hard to please my coaches and teachers so that I would receive from them the recognition that I needed. So, my father accomplished his goal, because of the way I responded. However, that is not the way I raised my children. I did praise them for doing a good job. I critiqued their work or play, but we always ended the conversation on a positive note.

With my father, there was no expressed appreciation for work well done. He had a very tough life. He had to work extremely hard to get by. He was very strict about what I could or could not do, and because I was successful in getting a college education and good paying job, he thought that he was successful. Therefore, he expected me to raise my children the same way I was raised. His attitude was that "It did not hurt you (me), so why was it not good enough for them?" When I was growing up at home and doing chores, I was expected to do every job correctly. If you did what you were told to do, "What was the big deal?" I can just imagine my dad saying, "Why should he expect a pat on the back? All he did was what he was supposed to do." You know, I think that is the way a lot of people believe today. As an employee or as a child, are you ever complimented for doing what you are told to do, or supposed to do? Usually not. However, for an employee or child to feel appreciated, they should be acknowledged for a job well done, even when it was part of their regular tasks. My father did not understand that it was necessary to express appreciation to someone for completing something even though it is simply part of their job.

Because there are no guarantees that we have any time except the present, we must take advantage of each opportunity we have to tell our friends and loved ones how much we appreciate them and love them. Many times, embarrassment will keep us from expressing our true feelings to a friend. I think men are particularly bad about this. As a man, we want to appear strong and "in control" to people. Being emotional does not fit that appearance. The "macho man" idea has made a lot of men hold back what their true emotions are, thus, those emotional words or feelings are never expressed. Each of us needs to get beyond this false ideology. There is no weakness in a man who cries. In fact, it is a strong man who can cry in front of others and not be embarrassed.

I was forty-eight years old before I ever defended myself to my father. Gwen was often frustrated with me, because I would not defend myself, nor her, when my father expressed his frustration with something that I did, or did not do. After his death, I found satisfaction in the fact that I had finally confronted my father that one Sunday afternoon when he was so furious about the picture collage. I took a stand for myself. By finally dealing with the problem, I felt better about myself. It felt good to take a stand for something I knew was right, but my father did not agree with. Why did it always have to be his narrow way of thinking? If I had not stood firm with him, I believe that I would have lived with regret that I never showed the courage to do so.

There is another aspect of my life with which I have no regrets. That is solely due to changes that occurred as a result of my cancer. In fact, I am proud of the fact that I can show my emotions in front of others today without being embarrassed. My emotions drastically changed after my first cancer diagnosis. I suddenly realized that I was not in control of my destiny. I needed help from my family, friends and those at work. It was not easy to admit that fact. The hardest thing that I had to do was go back to work following my first surgery. I knew that everyone at work had been informed that I had cancer and would be undergoing treatment. They would be expressing their care and concern to me. I anticipated that when they showed their compassion, I would not be able to control my emotions. Facing that was very difficult, but it was also very good for me to have to face that situation. My emotions have never been the same. If someone makes caring, kind, or loving comments about my children, or they show care for my children, I become teary-eyed very quickly. I was always a tenderhearted person, but my emotions have been greatly magnified since the cancer. I have become a very empathetic person. When someone else discusses life disappointments, I am right there in the same emotion with them. This is not something that I was comfortable with in the beginning, but I have become much more comfortable showing my emotions in front of others.

Chapter 17

Happiness in Life Is a Choice

"Be happy" or "be pessimistic"? What is **your** choice? This is a choice which each of us make in one way or another. Do you want others to view you as a person who usually has a smile on your face and enjoys life, or do you want others to recognize you as a person who always sees the worst in every situation?

If you care about how others categorize you, then there are certain things you should do to ensure that others have the correct impression of who you are. The most important thing is to approach every challenge with a positive attitude. It is easy to become discouraged when you are faced with disappointing news, but you can take that news and look for the positive things. If you are hearing some bad news, at least that means that you are still alive and able to think about its impact. Since you are alive and functioning mentally, that means that you still have the possibility to overcome the bad situation. It is possible that you recently suffered a major heart attack, or have been in a serious auto accident. You could have died instantly, but since you are reading this, that was not the case. You are alive and you have the opportunity to take care of some things that you may not have done yet. It may be a short time, but you have the privilege of some time—an opportunity to communicate those loving words that you have never made time to utter to your loved ones, or whatever has been lacking.

Maybe you need to apologize to someone. Take the opportunity to ease your conscience of anything that might be troubling you. If you are in this situation, take a minute to think about all of the people that you interact with on a regular basis. Are you quarrelling with anyone of those people right now? If so, do what is necessary to be at peace with that person. That will help you to reduce the stress in your life, plus you will be able to enjoy their friendship again. Is there someone in your family that you have "written off?" In other words, as far as you are concerned, they do not exist anymore. Hopefully that is not the case, but if it is, then be courageous and approach that person to let them know that you forgive them, or ask them for their forgiveness. Do whatever is necessary for you to be family once again. By mending the relationship, you will be relieved of that pain, plus they will not suffer when your time is over. When you find out that you are near the end of your life, or think that you may be, you may also find that you have more courage than ever before to deal with difficult situations. You may finally realize that the relational problems in your life should have never occurred in the first place, so it is time to make things right.

How do you view a challenging, disappointing or life-altering situation? Do you see it as another opportunity that God has given you to be an example to others, or do you ask, "Why me?" The way that a situation affects you, or should I say the way that you allow that situation to affect you, demonstrates the choice that you have already made. If you make the "choice" that you will strive to make the most (best) of every situation, you are making the choice to live a "happy life." That means that you will be looking for the positive results of an otherwise bad situation. If you look at each challenge in life as a struggle, or overwhelming burden that you do not want to deal with, then you are not going to be happy. In that case, life will be a very disappointing experience for you.

I am not about to tell you that I have handled every situation looking at it as an opportunity. However, I do believe that facing many different life-changing situations has made me a stronger person, who now looks for the positive more often. There will be times when you become overwhelmed and discouraged by what appears to be a "barrage" of bad circumstances that you have to face. But do not use that as a crutch! Just because it is probably going to happen, that does not mean that you should become discouraged and expect that it will usually be a negative experience. It does not have to be a negative result. Look for the positive things that can result from the situation.

My father happened to be a person who did not know how to look at the trying times as opportunities. It was very disheartening and frustrating to him, when his children or his grandchildren did not make the same choices that he would have made. He could only be happy and content with his family when they responded as he expected. The result of his lack of happiness was that family members did not want to share many life events with him. If my son or daughter had made a decision that I knew my father would not agree with, I would never share that with him. My children could have made a very good decision from which they prospered, but he would not agree.

We will be disappointed frequently, if we consistently place unrealistic expectations on our spouse or children. For example, if I expect my son to always make the same decision that I would have made in a situation, I am going to be disappointed each time that his decision is different than mine. It is unrealistic to expect another human being to always make the same choice that you would make. Instead, we need to recognize that there are several ways to accomplish a given task. As long as the task is accomplished without doing anything unethical or hurting anyone, then we should be pleased that the task was accomplished.

If you had a choice of either spending most of your time with a positive person or with a negative person, which would you choose? Most people prefer to be around individuals who are energetic and positive. If you want others to prefer to be around you, be sure that you exude happiness, joy and peace. Show others that you love life.

Chapter 18

Sharing Hope

You would never be faced with being personally impacted by an "act of God", a devastating calamity or loss of a loved one, if things were perfect. You would only deal with the natural process of losing those loved ones to old age. Unfortunately, most of us are not that lucky. Tragedy intercepts our regular routines when we least expect it. My family and I have personally experienced the trials detailed in this book. Hopefully, sharing my experiences in dealing with life's trials has given you insight that will help you deal with similar events that impact your life or the lives of those near and dear to you. My goal is that when you are confronted with a life-changing calamity, or someone is diagnosed with a serious disease, you will be armed with knowledge of lessons learned from real world situations, and that will allow you to better cope with the situation. If you are faced with a tragedy similar to one of my situations, you will know that others have faced this before, and survived. You can also realize that you do have a good chance of overcoming that adversity or disease, and be a stronger person for doing so.

By now you should be armed with valuable insight into ways to deal with your challenge at hand, or one that you may face in the future. Ideally, you are not in the middle of any crisis as you read this. Reading this book when you are in the middle of a disaster may, or may not, help you in dealing with that situation. When you are in the middle of a high-pressure ordeal, where everything seems to be working against you, it is very hard to find, or recognize, the positive things that are also occurring, or could result. It would be much more beneficial for you to read my book prior to facing any life-changing events. That is the ideal situation, but the book may not have reached you in time.

If I convey nothing else to you in this book, I would hope that you will seriously contemplate this one thought: When you are dealing with a life-changing situation that directly impacts you, do not ask God, "Why me? Why did you do this to me? Or, "What did I do to deserve this?" If you have a strong faith in God, do not let the diagnosis of a disease, or the occurrence of a life-changing misfortune cause you to lose your faith. Start "training your mind" with the thought that "If I am ever faced with having a serious disease or being part of a major disaster, I am not going to let go of my faith in God!" Times of great loss or harm are times when you need God the most. Do not blame God for the bad that comes upon you. God assures us that he will not allow us to be burdened with more trials and temptations than we are able to bear in I Corinthians 10:13 (KJV). God will provide a way of escape.

I Cor. 10:13 No temptation has overtaken you except such as is common to man; but God *is* faithful, who will not allow you to be tempted beyond what you are able, but with the temptation will also make the way of escape, that you may be able to bear *it*.

Furthermore, the New Testament assures us that God tempts no one in **James 1:13 (KJV).** We need to remember that the devil is tempting us, not God.

James 1:13 Let no one say when he is tempted, "I am tempted by God"; for God cannot be tempted by evil, nor does He Himself tempt anyone.

Look at the book of Job in the Old Testament. As you read chapters 1 and 2, you will see that God allowed Satan to tempt Job so long as he did not touch Job. Satan did the tempting. God did allow it to take place, but God did not tempt Job, nor will he tempt us. We have his promise on that.

You should prepare yourself to deal with tragedy, before you are in the middle of one. Speaking with God through prayer is the perfect avenue to keep this at the forefront of your thoughts. Ask God to give you the strength necessary to endure anything that comes your way. Pray that you will always be faithful to God and that your belief and trust in him will never waiver. Commit to yourself that you will NOT abandon your faith in times of distress or tragedy. Renew that commitment on a regular basis through prayer and positive thoughts of serving God. Remember the words of Paul in his first letter to the Thessalonians. Those words apply to us as well. In I Thess. 5:17 (KJV), Paul wrote "Pray without ceasing." If you keep spiritual thoughts at the forefront of your mind, you will have many less bad thoughts.

Maybe you do not want to think about negative situations. Personally, as I have grown older, I believe that I have grown to be more of a realist. I tend to look at things realistically, rather than just from a "positive" point of view. Do not get the wrong impression by that statement. I am a very positive thinking person and you should have seen that conveyed many times in my thoughts expressed in this book. Realistically, I know that at some point I am probably going to deal with another tragedy in my life, However, my philosophy is that if I have "programmed myself" to deal with a crisis by completely trusting in God, then I have a better chance of surviving the associated heartaches. I can grow stronger psychologically from the experience. I believe that each of us needs to "program self" so that we are prepared. When I say, "program self", I'm not talking about memorizing a series of phrases that emphasize the point, nor am I talking about repetition of catchy phrases to implant those phrases in your mind. It's a process of preparing yourself mentally and emotionally. Spend time meditating on a potential situation that you fear will happen to you. For example, "How am I going to survive if I lose one of my children?" Or maybe it is one of your parents or a good friend that is in poor health that you fear losing. Prepare yourself! While you are not faced with that kind of situation, think it through. Pray to God for the strength and guidance to get you through the tough times. Try to identify what will give you the most strength to make it through. Is it the Bible? If your answer is "Yes", make a commitment to yourself that you will turn to the Bible. If you are lacking a good Bible study or Bible reading habit right now, start developing one. Open the Bible each day and read a short message from God's Word.

Is one of your weaknesses that you normally withdraw from everyone around you when a troubling situation occurs? If that is your typical response, you need to promise yourself that you are not going to withdraw from those close to you; that you will stay involved with them. Make a commitment to yourself that you will seek help from friends, family and loved ones. Or, you may address the "programming" in a more generic sense. Just contemplate what you will do if you are faced with a life-changing event. You do not have to identify a specific situation, but think through what you must always do when confronted with a trying time. Think about situations in the past where you were dealing with a tough ordeal. What could you have done differently that would have helped you? For a spiritually minded person, on top of everything else you do, always remember to pray to God in trying times. Speaking with God and trusting in Him can ease your burden.

Keeping things in the proper perspective is difficult when you are faced with bad news. We get so caught up in fear and remorse that we forget about all the good in our life. I hope that the "programming" or "preparing yourself" concept makes practical sense to you. Being caught totally off-guard with a tough situation can be overwhelming. Even when you are prepared, it can still be overwhelming, so the better prepared you are, the less stress you will experience.

Here is another recommendation. The next time a small problem occurs, practice sharing your burdens with someone you know very well. That may be someone at church; a close family member, or a good friend. You know who you can confide in. Seek out that person. In the Bible, we read:

Gal. 6:2 Bear ye one another's burdens, and so fulfill the law of Christ.

We are instructed to help each other by sharing the burden. That is hard to do if you do not know that someone is dealing with a heavy burden. You need to help others to help you by sharing your troubles with them. Many times when you are struggling through a tough situation, your friends ask, "Is there anything that I can do for you?" The typical response is "No thanks, I am fine" or, "It is not that big a deal." If it is not that big a deal, then why are you totally consumed with the thought of it? Why does it cause you to be so depressed, if it is not a big deal? We do not want to be a burden to anyone else with our problems, so we do not let them into our lives. If those friends are like me, when they ask that question of someone, they really want to help you. However, if you will not be open with your friend and talk about the tough situation at hand, there is not much that your friend can do for you. I want to encourage you to respond to that question of "Is there anything that I can do for you?" with a very clear request for help like, "I would like for you to say a prayer with me," or "It would sure be nice if you would drop my clothes off at the cleaners." Giving your friends an opportunity to help you is fulfilling for them. Think about what you have just read! It is fulfilling to those that want to help you. Wow! It is not all about you. You are actually helping someone dear to you when you let him or her share your pains; your trials, and your grief. I feel honored and humbled when someone feels comfortable enough with me to share their troubles and ask me for specific help.

Has there been a situation where you had a troubled friend and you were able to do a little something for them? How did that make you feel? Good? Worthwhile? Like I stated before, it is very rewarding to me when I am able to help someone. Let your friends experience that same feeling, by letting them help you. This is an area where I have changed. Years ago, when someone would ask, "Can I help in any way?" I would reply "No thanks." But today, if a person asks a question like that, I assume that they are sincere when they ask, and if there is something that I need, I will let them know. It is their problem if they were being insincere when they asked the question. You can also tell by their response to your request if they were sincere, or not. If you ask for help, then they start stuttering and making excuses; you know that they did not really want to help. That is rare, but it can happen. When you recognize that insincerity, you can let them off the hook by telling them, "It is no big deal. Do not worry about it."

When our house was flooded, there were only three families in our small neighborhood whose homes were not flooded. One of those families suffered from the guilt they felt, because they were not flooded. They felt guilty, while I felt that they were very lucky and I was happy that they did not suffer the same problems. Was it their fault that their house was not flooded? No way! To help them overcome those guilty feelings, that family was compelled to help those of us who were victims. They opened their house to everyone so people could use their bathroom, or stop by and rest. They provided meals and ran errands for others. Now I ask you— how would they have worked through their guilty feelings if when they offered help, everyone replied, "No thanks, we can handle the issues ourselves."? They could have taken that kind of response as "You have no idea what it is like to be flooded", or venting of anger because they escaped the disaster. They would have felt helpless and even more guilty. You might be amazed at how much good you are doing for others when you allow them to help you.

Believe me, when I say that I understand that it is difficult to acknowledge that you need help the first time. It is just as hard to ask someone close to you for help when you need it, especially that first time that help is needed. When I was diagnosed with cancer the first time, I dreaded my return to work. I recognized that I was going to need others to cover for me at work when I was not feeling well following a treatment. I also knew that I needed their encouragement. Things were out of my control for the first time in my life. I did not know what the next six months would involve as I went through the chemotherapy. But, you know what? Everyone was anxious and more than willing to help me. It provided them with an opportunity to reach out and help someone. I was not the burden that I was afraid that I would be.

I truly hope that you have found comforting, helpful points from the experiences that have been shared in this book. Thank you for allowing me to share just a part of my life. If and when you are faced with a life-altering calamity, I encourage you to deal with it head on by accepting your current circumstances, and ask God to help you make it through the difficult challenges ahead. Remember, "With God, all things are possible." **Matthew 19:26; Mark 10:27 (KJV)**

Chapter 19

Our Lives Today

Our lives have been extremely blessed in the last few years. Todd graduated from college in December, 2005. Garrett's graduation was in May 2006 and Whitney will finish her Bachelor's degree in December. Both of our sons were able to find good jobs immediately following college. In 1993, I had prayed to live long enough to watch my children walk the stage at their high school graduation. As of today, I have been able to enjoy so much more. Garrett was our first child to be married this summer, following his graduation, and we love his wife, Kelly, a wonderful addition to our family. Todd is soon to be engaged to Lindsay, and we can hardly wait. If it is God's will, we will enjoy many more happy occasions together as a family.

In 2004, Gwen and I became associates of the #1 network marketing company, which manufactures pharmaceutical grade supplements. We focus on using optimal nutrition for controlling my cancer, and maintaining our health. Through our relationship with this unique company, we have been introduced to a holistic approach to healthcare. I have entrusted my physical life to Sanoviv Medical Institute, where world-class doctors treat you using a comprehensive program that focuses on the mind, body and soul. Don't get me wrong. I still see my oncologist every six months for blood work and have a CT-scan annually to ensure that my good health continues. But, I have great confidence that if my cancer were to reappear, I have connected myself with a medical facility that can treat my disease successfully. My goal is to attend Sanoviv annually.

Gwen has found her much needed financial security as an Independent Associate. She is very passionate about the opportunity that she has to enrich the lives and health of thousands of people. And, we enjoy working with our family, our long-time friends, and the many new friends who have joined our business, because we know that it will provide them with good health and a solid residual income.

After any visit with family members, or when ending a phone conversation, I make sure that I voice "I love you" before we part. I don't want to miss an opportunity to express my love for them. As you can see, I am living a full, blessed life for which I am extremely grateful.

Printed in the United States
66597LVS00001B/151-273